Praise for *Scaling Force...*

"I love this book! I like the authors as people and I highly recommend all their work. However, I have to say that I think this book is my favourite. It's my favourite because it superbly addresses what I feel is the biggest problem in modern self-defence training; namely that far too many people think that self-protection is the same as martial arts, is the same as fighting. Don't get me wrong, I love the martial arts and I enjoy a good spar in the dojo, but it's a big mistake to think that they give you all you need to protect yourself from violence.

"Whenever I tell people that they should be careful not to confuse martial arts and fighting for self-protection, the common reaction is for them to get all bent out of shape and tell me how effective their style of fighting is. What they fail to grasp is that you could be studying an amazingly effective system of fighting, but self-protection is not about fighting. I know some great fighters who are piss-poor when it comes to defending themselves. They end up in fights all the time, some have ended up in jail, and three are missing body parts (two ears, one finger, and a testicle overall). Are they effective fighters? Sure! Were their self-protection skills effective? Nope!

"Put it this way, would you learn road safety from the guy who said, 'I've been ran over by one thousand cars and I survived every one!' This is what we see all the time in self-protection training though: the equivalent of people teaching how to roll over car bonnets (that should be 'hoods' in the US right?) and passing that off as all you need to know about road safety. Sure, self-protection has a physical component, but it's a massive mistake to take that one part and believe it to be the whole. Even the physical side of self-protection is not the same as a 'fight,' but let's park that for now.

"If you are serious about learning self-protection, and not indulging some testosterone fuelled, celluloid inspired fantasy, then you need a much wider skill set than most appreciate.

"You need to know the law, and in my experience here in the UK most instructors misunderstand the law to the point where they terrify their students into inaction or make them jailbirds in waiting.

"You need to know how physical conflict can be avoided, and in my experience most simply say 'avoid fights if you can—and having said that let's get back to how to rip windpipes out.' There are skills associated with avoiding violence and, in my view, they are far more important to acquire than a powerful right cross: lip service is not enough. It's a pet peeve of mine when I see 'self-defence' books and courses begin with "Lesson 1: How to get out of a headlock." They should back up a bit and look at the whole chain of events that lead to them being in the headlock. If you don't have the skills to stop situations before they develop into physical violence guess what you're going to experience a lot of? Self-protection is about keeping ourselves safe, right?

"You need to be able to use the right tools for the circumstances. There is an old saying, 'When all you have is a hammer, then every problem is a nail.' If fighting is all you have, then that's going to be your solution to everything, whether it is applicable or not. Is that punch to the throat really what you need to deal with a drunk relative at wedding? (I'm assuming drunken family brawls happen as commonly at US weddings as they do at UK ones.) Are you really going to try to reason with a person who is being unreasonable? I once witnessed a training course where the instructor advised trying to calm a person down when they were already throwing punches. Not a good idea! You need to be able to use the tools and skills most applicable to the circumstances; and you can't do that if you can't read the circumstances or you don't have those tools. This book can help fix that.

"As I read the book what struck me was how similar this was to how the UK police force are trained. And the reason they are trained to cover all of the topics herein is because that's what they need to effectively address conflict and violence as it really is. Many martial artists and 'self-defence instructors' work backward and reinvent violence to fit their 'pre-existing solution.' However, the only way to be effectively prepared is to look at the reality of the situation and forge a solution from there. Anyone and any group who does that will find their answers will be as presented herein.

"I feel this has to be the most thorough presentation of true self-protection out there. The knowledge contained within is what anybody who is serious about keeping himself safe needs to know. I hope the book is as massively successful as it deserves to be and that in doing so it busts once and for all the myth that martial arts and fighting are one and the same as self-protection."

—*Iain Abernethy, 6th Dan, British Combat Association Hall of Fame Member* (www.iainabernethy.com)

~~~

"When it comes to using your self-defense training you only have two problems. One is if it doesn't work. Two is if it does work. Both can get you into serious trouble. This book is for keeping you out of the second kind of trouble. A raw and horrible truth is most of what you think you know about self-defense is advertising, if not an outright lie. The biggest myth is that self-defense is a martial art, MMA or combatives term. It's not. It is a legal term. It is those standards you will be held accountable to. You'll not be judged according to what you were told in training nor what you heard on an internet forum filled with cyber-warriors, 'well I would have' studs and there-are-no-rules-in-a-street-fight commandos. Your actions will be judged by legal standards. Both Miller and Kane have hundreds of hands-on violent encounters under their belts. They understand the importance of knowing the legal restrictions of force, how to judge the danger, how to choose the right response level, how to articulate those choices, and how to navigate the trap-filled aftermath of violence. Information they share with you in this book will keep you from going to prison for 'defending' yourself."

—*Marc MacYoung* (www.nononsenseselfdefense.com)

~~~

"There are two aspects of self-defense training that are sorely lacking, in my experience. But first, let me ask you a question: if I told you I was opening a driving school, but the only aspects of driving I would concentrate on would be proper turning of the steering wheel, shifting gears, pedal control, seatbelts, use of mirrors and the like, while disregarding things like what side of the road to drive on, the speed limit, right of way, and the other legalities that make driving from Point A to Point B possible, would you think I was crazy? Yet this happens every day in martial arts training across the world—students being taught every aspect of the mechanics of their art, all the moves, katas, forms, etc., yet not being taught that things like laws can limit or allow certain actions. If you win the fight but end up in prison, did you really win? No one would learn to drive a car from someone who doesn't teach traffic laws, but instructors do it all the time in the martial arts. So think of this book as an excellent general introduction to figuring out what side of the road you can drive on. It will be an eye-opener.

"Secondly, imagine that not only did you not learn about traffic laws, but the very first time you drove was having to drive a family member to the emergency room at rush hour, in an ice storm. That's a steep learning curve, and make no mistake: That's also what a critical incident can feel like, when all of your martial training, learned in the comfort and safety of the *dojo*, might as well be quantum physics for your ability to utilize it. I can't tell you what your first fight, or first self-defense scenario, or your first critical incident will be like. No one can. What I can tell you, as an officer with two decades-long law enforcement, is the one immutable law I know of this type of events—your next incident won't be what you think it'll be. It may not even be close. So it's best to cover as many bases as you can in your training.

"This book is one of the best I've read, and I've read most of them, about what you may encounter in the self-defense domain and the challenges you'll face. Miller and Kane have been there, done that, and have the t-shirt. And they're giving you their lessons learned without requiring you to pay the fee in blood like they had to in order to learn them. And that is priceless."

—*M. Guthrie, Federal Air Marshal*

~~~

"As a martial art and self-defense instructor, who is also a licensed attorney, I'm often concerned with self-defense classes, courses, books, and DVDs that neglect the importance of teaching legal ramifications of violence along with the physical principles and techniques to hurt another human being. I also notice the absence, or minimal instruction, of topics such as awareness, avoidance, de-escalation, and levels of force. Not every situation calls for the 'kill 'em all, let God sort them out' response. And the flippant, 'I'd rather be tried by twelve than carried by six' while true, doesn't help when you are in prison. Finally, Miller and Kane have written a book that provides much more than a cursory look at some very important elements regarding
~~~

violence. *Scaling Force* doesn't only provide tools on how to deal with violence, but when and to what level you should deal with violence. The combined knowledge will not only keep you safe and alive, but out of prison. Personally, I don't want to be tried or carried, and the information in this book can help you avoid both, or at the very least, if tried, you can prevail in that arena too. Students of martial arts and self-defense should study this closely, and instructors should incorporate these lessons into their teaching. If you don't, you are doing your students a disservice by not teaching everything that belongs in a self-defense course. Miller and Kane have written a great addition to everyone's self-defense library."

—*Alain Burrese, Attorney, Author, Former US Army sniper* (www. burrese.com)

~~~

"Miller and Kane have done a tremendous service for instructors like myself. They have written, in a clear, thoughtful, provocative, and undeniably profound manner, a book that teaches people what they need to know BEFORE they get into a fight and what they need to know if they cannot extricate themselves from one. This is an incredible book that I will insist all my martial arts and firearms students read. I always recommend *On Killing*, but I think this book is even better for these purposes as it is all about living in a civilian world. It will undoubtedly save lives and hopefully much anguish."

—*Ron Breines, Kyoshi—Kakuto Ryu Jujutsu/Karate-Jutsu, certified firearms/self-defense tactical instructor*

~~~

"When Rory and Lawrence asked me to publicly share my thoughts on *Scaling Force*, I was both honored and a little hesitant at the prospect. Anyone familiar with the work of these two men, as writers, teachers, and professionals, knows they speak (and act) plainly, frankly and, perhaps most importantly to someone like me, from hard experience. In my estimation, they wrote *Scaling Force* in this manner. In the proper hands, this book will serve the reader as a guide to help select, employ, and articulate a level of physical force appropriate to a given situation—from sparring in a training hall, to preventing cranky ol' Uncle Dutch from driving home drunk, to fighting for your life at the hands of an assailant.

"Ironically, this brings me to the 'hesitation' I mentioned: As competent and well-written as *Scaling Force* is, it's only a guide, albeit a really good one. Rory and Lawrence make no bones about this fact, warning the reader that in order to successfully apply the knowledge to be gained from this book, you have to know what to practice, why you need to practice, and then you actually have to practice. You must set aside any fantasies you may have about how applying force to another person—or having him (or them) apply it to you—looks, feels, smells, and can affect you for the rest of your life. You can't just read, mull over, or mentally rehearse (although mental rehearsal certainly has its value); you have to get up and move. In my experience, most people aren't willing to adopt this mindset or subject themselves to the sort of discomfort (physical and psychological) it demands. Yet I wonder how many of them will read this work and find a way to weave its information into even more intricate fantasies.

"I hope I'm wrong and that the vast majority of readers will instead put the authors' collective skill and experience to good use. If you're serious about learning how the application of physical force works—before, during, and after the fact—I cannot recommend this book highly enough."

—*Lieutenant Jon Lupo, New York State Police*

~~~

"Rory and Lawrence make their position on violence quite clear: Avoid it. When you can. But then while most of us civilians don't intentionally face off with angry drunks or get jumped by ninja wannabes, there may be moments when we have no choice but to make a decision. In this book, two of the mellowest guys I know address this decision spectrum. When do you walk away from an insult, try to talk down the angry drunk, take a baseball bat to an intruder, shoot an armed robber? Do you have to be the victim to take action? Can you go to jail for that? Clearly the use of force is not as TV would have us believe. With exercises and anecdotes, *Scaling Force* explores the motivations, the decision spectrum, and the consequences, because there are always consequences. Don't confuse mellow with wimpy; Rory and Lawrence have been there, and they tell their stories well."

—*Julie Van Dielen, Law Enforcement Training Resources*
(www.letrainingresources.com)

~~~

"*Scaling Force* is a scholarly, yet highly readable text, jam-packed with the crucial elements needed to survive a brutal attack. This is unique and vital information that too many instructors don't teach or don't know. Let Miller and Kane, two veterans of countless down-and-dirty confrontations, give you the edge to survive a dangerous situation."

—*Loren W. Christensen, 8th dan black belt, author* (www.lwcbooks.com)

~~~

"Miller/Kane have yet again provided law-abiding citizens with the tools to truly protect themselves. While instruction on the mechanics and techniques of self-defense and deadly force is readily available from multiple sources, this book gives you so much more. Miller/Kane provide the reader with the 'big picture' of a deadly force incident which goes so much further than the split-second physical incident. The aftermath of such an incident is often as 'life threatening' as the moment itself. The emotional and financial stresses resulting from use of force can be absolutely devastating. I cannot recommend this book enough. Take advantage of the information compiled from hundreds of case studies to better prepare yourself if the day comes when you have to make that 'life-changing' decision."

—*Tracy Getty, Certified Firearms Instructor*
~~~

SCALING FORCE

DYNAMIC DECISION MAKING UNDER THREAT OF VIOLENCE

SCALING FORCE

DYNAMIC DECISION MAKING UNDER THREAT OF VIOLENCE

Understand

How to stop violence before it happens

How to choose the right response level

How to avoid going to jail for defending yourself

by
Rory Miller
&
Lawrence A. Kane

YMAA Publication Center, Inc.
Wolfeboro NH USA

YMAA Publication Center, Inc.
PO Box 480
Wolfeboro, NH 03894
800-669-8892 • www.ymaa.com • info@ymaa.com

Paperback
ISBN: 978-1-59439-250-4

Ebook
ISBN: 978-1-59439-251-1

Cover design by Axie Breen
Editing by Susan Bullowa
Photos by Lawrence A. Kane unless noted otherwise.

POD0916

Publisher's Cataloging in Publication

Miller, Rory.

Scaling force : dynamic decision making under threat of violence / by Rory Miller & Lawrence A. Kane. – Wolfeboro, NH : YMAA Publication Center, c2012.

p. ; cm.

ISBN: 978-1-59439-250-4 (pbk.) ; 978-1-59439-251-1 (ebk.)
"Understand how to stop violence before it happens, how to choose the right response level, how to avoid going to jail for defending yourself."
Includes bibliographical references and index.

1. Violence – Prevention – Handbooks, manuals, etc. 2. Self-defense – Handbooks, manuals, etc. 3. Violence – Psychological aspects. 4. Martial arts – Handbooks, manuals, etc. 5. Fighting (Psychology) 6. Self-defense (Law) – United States. I. Kane, Lawrence A. (Lawrence Alan) II. Title. III. Title: Dynamic decision-making under threat of violence.

GV1102.7.P75 M557 2012
613.6/6–dc23 1110

Warning: While self-defense is legal, fighting is illegal. If you don't know the difference you'll go to jail because you aren't defending yourself, you are fighting—or worse. Readers are encouraged to be aware of all appropriate local and national laws relating to self-defense, reasonable force, and the use of weaponry, and to act in accordance with all applicable laws at all times. Understand that while legal definitions and interpretations are generally uniform, there are small—but very important—differences from state to state and even city to city. To stay out of jail, you need to know these differences. Neither the authors nor the publisher assumes any responsibility for the use or misuse of information contained in this book.

Nothing in this document constitutes a legal opinion nor should any of its contents be treated as such. While the authors believe that everything herein is accurate, any questions regarding specific self-defense situations, legal liability, and/or interpretation of federal, state, or local laws should always be addressed by an attorney at law. This text relies on public news sources to gather information on various crimes and criminals described herein. While news reports of such incidences are generally accurate, they are on occasion incomplete or incorrect. Consequently, all suspects should be considered innocent until proven guilty in a court of law.

When it comes to martial arts, self-defense, and related topics, no text, no matter how well written, can substitute for professional, hands-on instruction. These materials should be used **for academic study only**.

Printed in USA.

DEDICATION

Dedicated to the memory of Tim Bown (1977–2010), Bulletman extraordinaire. A good man, a good friend, a good father, and a good husband. You will be missed, brother. See you on the other side.

CONTENTS

ACKNOWLEDGMENTS

Our gratitude to martial arts instructor Mauricio Machuca for sharing his experience of what it's like to be on the wrong end of a knife encounter and to Federal Air Marshal M. Guthrie for providing insight into the effects of adrenaline on performance in combat. Thanks to Joey Kane, Chris Nunez, Adriana Tabile, Hazel Tabile, Natalia Tabile, and Raul Tabile for braving near arctic conditions to be stars in our photos. Also thanks to Sonia Lyris who not only starred in our pics but helped direct them as well. Much appreciated. Y'all rock!

For practical skills and applications, the list is long. Ron Bishop and Paul McRedmond for early training in ethically applying force: "You can do the right thing or the safe thing. We're sworn to do the right thing." *Sensei* Dave Sumner and *Sensei* Kris Wilder who taught new worlds of physical skills. Small Circle JJ instructor Stan Miller who taught stuff that made handcuffing much easier. Hundreds of officers, martial artists, and training partners, and thousands of crooks all of whom taught invaluable lessons. Thanks!

FOREWORD—CLINT OVERLAND

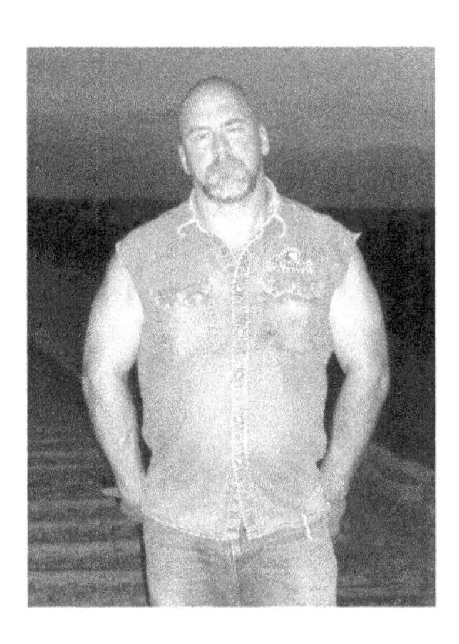

Clint Overland spent 22 years as a bouncer, thug, and SOB for hire. Not someone you want hanging around your teenage sons as a role model. Reformed, he currently lives in West Texas with his beautiful wife and four children, two dogs, three cats, and four guinea pigs. He's trying to make up for some of the bad he has done by telling people the truth about training for real violence. You can reach him at coverland69@suddenlink.net

Let me start by telling a short story just to set the theme. The job was to find a guy who had made a friend of their boss mad. They were to hurt the individual bad enough for him to understand that he had crossed a line that should not even have been approached. The target was known to the two breakers and they took turns watching, learning his pattern and habits for several days. Come Friday night, they were waiting for him at the local tavern where he stopped for a drink after work. The target came in, had several beers, and walked into the restroom. The breakers followed him and while one watched the door, the larger one approached the target who was taking a leak. Slamming the target's face into the top of the urinal, knocking out all of his teeth, the breaker began stomping on the target's prone body, over and over again. The target was left alive, most of his ribs, both of his collar bones, one arm, and one leg broken into multiple pieces. For their work, the breakers were given a one thousand dollar bonus each.

What's the difference in the actions of the two breakers and what is being taught in today's *dojos* and training halls? The breakers weren't there to earn a point, gain a belt, or follow some system of honor. No, they were there to do a job and get paid for it. They are professionals and they went about their job as quickly and proficiently as possible. No ego boosting, no getting worked up and adrenalized. They simply took care of business.

Professional violence is a business and one that I am well acquainted with!

I spent twenty-two years working as a bouncer and as a problem solver like the breakers above. I have seen the absolute worst that humans can and often do to each other. Sadly, in another life, I was more than willing to do the exact same thing. One therapist, right before he fired me as his patient told me, and I quote, "You were born a mean tempered son-of-a-bitch and I don't think I can help you anymore!" Another one said I was a "functioning sociopath with mid-level psychotic tendencies" and that I gave him nightmares so he couldn't see me again. I started noticing a pattern after that...

So when I discuss violence, its cause, effects, and outcomes, I know just enough to make myself somewhat understood. I am not a martial artist nor do I teach any self-defense class. I am a reformed knee-breaker and professional thug. The book you're holding in your hands is a book about violence. Not some glorified Hollywood version of a violence-junkie's masturbation scene but real violence that often leads to prison or death.

A lot of the time I find myself laughing at some of the things I see on YouTube and other internet sites; I mean, come on people, where do you come up with this stuff? I don't argue the point that picking someone up and smashing his head onto the concrete isn't effective;

it's also attempted murder. Think I am kidding? Watch a couple of the more popular self-defense videos and you will see what I mean. If you're *that* mad at someone, put a zip-tie around his neck, jerk it tight, then sit back and watch. It's a lot easier and makes for a better show.

Another thing I find funny is the way some of the stuff I see advertised is simply ineffective and really dangerous to the once-a-week practitioner. I am no martial artist; the last thing I want to do is get into a fight with you. Slip behind you and beat you down with a hammer maybe. Fight you? Hell no, I might get hurt!

Let me tell you another story and maybe you will start to understand. I was working at a college bar in Lubbock, Texas. Nice little place where the frat boys like to come and tear stuff up, and pay for damages with daddy's money. I was enjoying the scenery; it was a real "how slutty can I get away with" night, when one of the regulars, a juice monkey (steroid abuser), walked up to me. I'm six-foot-four and weigh around 260 to 270 lbs. This guy dwarfed me by about four inches and was shredded like a poster boy for a chemical awareness ad (I swear he was one injection away from a nuclear meltdown). He starts telling me about how he won a shot at some MMA tournament coming up in a few months. I told him congratulations and wished him the best. We talked for a little while and enjoyed the boobs walking by. He went on to hang out with some friends and I thought everything was good. I was wrong!

About an hour later Juice Boy walks up to me and starts telling me how he could take me. I said, "Bro, in a ring you would beat me to death. I'm no MMA fighter; hell, I am not even involved in the martial arts." Juice Boy then spouts off, "No I could take you right here!" Now I am watching him start to swell up, nostrils flaring, and real stupid ideas swarming through his head. I know I have to end this quick or I will be shitting teeth and pissing blood come the morning and I hate that. So I snap my hand out and poke him in the eye with my index finger, sink it in about a half an inch. He hits the ground screaming, I simply ask him, "What, didn't you hear the bell?"

I guess I said that to get to this: I am not playing by your rules. Yes, there are rules, even in a street fight, no matter what you thought you knew. One of the big ones is "Don't kill the other guy." Another,

"Don't get caught." What, you think that those aren't rules? They are, and they're big ones. Your anal virginity is depending on them! Unless prison rape sounds like a grand idea, then be my guest and break them. Lots of people thought they knew what self-defense was 'till they had to explain their actions to a jury.

I really should be mad as hell at Miller and Kane. I mean, come on guys, who needs a book telling you how to survive a run-in with a professional criminal? You should just keep your head buried in the sand and drink the Kool-Aid that your twenty-one-year-old 4th degree karate master tells you. Hell, that's what you are paying him a $150.00 dollars a month for isn't it? You don't need to know that the killer MMA moves you learned last week will land you in prison doing the shower-shuffle with Bubba and Earl do you? No, and you shouldn't have to worry about meeting someone that just plain don't give a fuck about you and gets his rocks off by bashing your brains out your nose! And who in their right mind would ever think that when they stomp the guy that took a swing at them, that it wasn't self-defense?

I wish I'd had this book when I started. Would have saved me a small fortune on lawyers and bail bondsmen! But, besides that, it might have given me the foresight and knowledge so that I could still chew on both sides.

In the following pages, you will find a complete school on what to do and what not to do. Certain misconceptions and outright fantasies will be shattered for some. Others will find a few open-mouth face-slaps—"Why didn't I think of it that way" moments. And you will really start to see and comprehend why self-defense isn't always what you think it is.

Don't just read this book, study it. Think about what the authors are trying to get across to you. Go through it again and again until it sinks in. Work the drills and practice the techniques they discuss. This book could honestly save your life and the life of your loved ones, because you aren't the only one to suffer when you go to prison. I know too many guys that are doing time because they thought they knew some form of martial art and had a small understanding of the justice system, that they could get away with pounding someone's head in during a bar fight. Reality is a major bitch especially when you get to court and are cleared of criminal charges only to have the other guy serve you for civil court as you walk out.

Miller and Kane really have been there and done that; it's not a fun place to be. When your entire livelihood and future depends on the whim of twelve people that weren't smart enough to get out of jury duty, needless to say it causes a little stress! Every lawyer who deals in self-defense cases needs to read this book. It may help them keep their client out of prison, so buy another copy and send it to an attorney too!

Let me give you a few more reasons to really study and pay attention to what Miller and Kane are trying to get across to you. I don't get sick anymore. Funny reason, huh? The smell of fresh-spilt intestines doesn't bother me. Neither does trying to hold them in place while their owner writhes around, screaming. All because he mouthed off to the wrong Mexican, who didn't play by middle-class white boy rules. The smell of someone's brain's laying on the ground doesn't faze me either; funny I think they smell like Ivory soap. Sick, I know, but they really do!

There are a lot worse out there than me and they don't care what "Über-ninja badass martial art" you practice. They don't care where you study, what you know, or who you are. They will split your gut open from your balls to your brisket without blinking an eye. And you will never see it coming.

I really think that's what Miller and Kane are trying to get across to you in this book; it's not always what it appears to be. The key word is "it." It is the ideas that you have formed from television, movies, the internet, and other media. It is the miscomprehensions and false sense of reality that come from training and studying under someone who doesn't understand the facts himself. And in most cases doesn't even know it.

I remember a case in Dallas several years ago where a woman was attacked by her husband. She had been studying Krav Maga. And *she* was the one to go to the penitentiary for attempted murder. Why you ask? After her husband was down, she proceeded to stomp him in the testicles and head, even after he was unconscious. This is what her teacher had trained her to do. Well, sorry but after he was no longer a threat, he became the victim. It's that easy to screw up and ruin your life in a matter of moments.

Like I said before, don't just read this book, but study it. Learn it and apply the ideas and principles taught to your martial arts training or self-defense portfolio. If you still think it's really not that important, you need to pay close attention to my last few statements.

If and, I hope not when, you get into an altercation with another individual, then every aspect of your life will be on trial. Every statement or post on your social networking site. Every martial arts/self-defense class you have ever taken. Everything you have ever done will be scrutinized and examined by the District/Prosecuting Attorney. It can and will be used against you in ways that you never thought possible. If by some chance, you are found not-guilty, then be prepared for the lawyers in the civil case that is coming to play even dirtier than the D.A. Your character, reputation, family history, everything about you and yours, will be on display for the jury and world to see. Think it is a joke? Talk to someone that has been through it and you will find out just how bad it can be.

FOREWORD — RON BISHOP

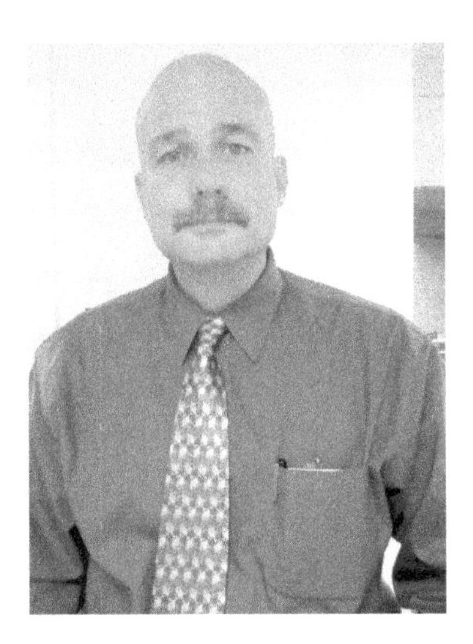

Ron Bishop has been in Law Enforcement/Corrections for the past 27 years. He is an established and recognized expert in police/ corrections use of force, deadly force, and logistical operations. Ron has served as a command level officer with his agency for the past 15 years, advising and establishing policy and practices. He has testified in both Federal and State level cases involving force and operational issues. Ron is a graduate of the National Institute of Corrections Leadership and Executive programs and holds the highest level of certifications in the State of Oregon. He is an active Freemason. Ron resides in the State of Washington with his wife and two daughters.

Those who just put this book down are risking everything, maybe even their freedom.

When violence comes to you, will you survive? I would bet that several who just read that question replied "Yes."

Let me pose a question to you: Have you ever considered that your training can be used against you? I am not speaking about a physical altercation but in a court of law.

How would you respond when asked by plaintiff's counsel, "You have martial arts training, correct?"

And you say, "Yes."

Then you are asked, "Your training covers various techniques ranging from simple moves all the way to complex moves that can cause significant injury, correct?"

And you respond, "Well it's more than that."

And then the golden question is brought to you: "You are taught control in class, correct? To strike without hurting. Correct?"

You just look at the attorney like a deer in the headlights not wanting to be there. Now he goes for your throat, turns to the jury and asks, "Why would anyone with your skill and training need to use so much force on a person like my client who does not have this same training?"

Just get out your checkbook because it's going to be a poor day for you.

Does that really happen? I will tell you, yes. It does. Having been involved in a fight that lasted over six minutes with extreme violence and ended with deadly results, I was asked similar questions. My vast law enforcement training ranging from communication training to physical defensive tactics were analyzed by the plaintiff's counsel. The incident I was involved in resulted in no criminal indictments but an out-of-court cash settlement due to evidence that the federal judge disallowed.

The Sheriff said, "You used your knowledge and training to control a horribly out-of-control inmate. The settlement was about our chances in court."

We survived criminal liability by being reviewed (testifying) in front of a grand jury. We survived civil liability because we acted within the scope of our jobs, we did not overreact, and we followed the law. The civil settlement still bothers me today because we did nothing wrong and used our training.

There are three golden rules that are the mantra in most law-enforcement training classes when dealing with use of force situations:

- Go home safe.
- The bad guy goes/stays in jail.
- Liability free.

As a training officer, I have said these rules. As a student of Rory Miller, I have heard these rules in almost every class. In this book, Miller and Kane will teach you how to respond in a manner that may increase your chances of surviving a multitude of situations.

Have you ever considered the potential limitations of your martial arts or self-defense training? In no manner am I suggesting that martial arts training or self-defense classes are bad. I am cautioning that an important element may be missing in your training. This book aids the reader in developing potential knowledge to close that gap.

In the classes that I have instructed or in the review process when conferring with attorneys, I ask the question: "Is every use of force situation the same?" The answer is no. Force situations are like games of chess; no two are alike unless reenacted. There are so many variables to consider when responding to a situation.

Before we go further, let me pose a question: Is controlled training (studio) the same as a necessary response in an uncontrolled environment? Let me respond with this answer. My wife is a better target shooter with a firearm then I am, but I am a better combat shooter. In her world (no disrespect), she has time to sight, she understands time, the rules, and what end result is desired. In the world of combat, the variables are constantly changing to include...everything. It's the chess analogy.

When violence comes to you, how will you react? If you overreact, as defined by the courts, you lose. You may lose your house, possessions, and freedom. All because you acted as you were trained. You could also under-react, and end up dead.

There are conditioned responses in some training that cause a person to increase, decrease, or even stop what they are doing.

Other responses are to continue until your opponent is no longer a threat. Either conditioning can lead to a bad end result. Reacting too small can get you hurt. Acting too harsh may land you in court. This book helps you find the area where you are most comfortable.

When dealing with force, there is the art of disengagement. You may ask, "What, run away?" My response is yes. Years ago a trooper from the state where I reside stopped a car and upon exiting his patrol car, four bad guys got out of the stopped vehicle with bats and sticks. The trooper was told to get back in his car and he would not be harmed. How did the trooper respond? He disengaged. The bad guys left. About four miles down the road, the trooper stopped the vehicle again, with backup. A lot of backup. Nobody got hurt, bad guys went to jail, and the incident was liability free. The trooper may have been justified to shoot at the four bad guys, but chose a different force option. Think about it.

In another example, a friend of mine was a recruit 25 years ago and saw what he described as "the shit monster in a beater car give him the finger." He attempted a car stop, but the monster drove to his home. Once home, the monster got out of the car and started walking toward a shed that had chain saws and swing blades. My friend then saw four younger versions of the monster who had given him the finger walking toward him. He told me, "I thought someone was going to die over giving me the finger?" He disengaged. How would court have gone for him if he had not?

For the past 17 years of my 27-year career, I have had the responsibility of reviewing use of force reports looking for policy violations, state law violations, and liability issues. During that period of time, I have reviewed uncountable reports from Miller. I never sent a situation that he handled for investigation. Further I know that he has defused situations ranging from a drunken idiot to an inmate with a shank. I have served with him in numerous venues and have found him to be a sound operative.

Miller and Kane have taken their experience both in law enforcement and martial arts, and have created a book that should cause a reader to pause and think about a proper response to a given situation.

When violence comes to you, will you survive? Many have, many didn't. Many wish they did.

Stay safe.

—RB

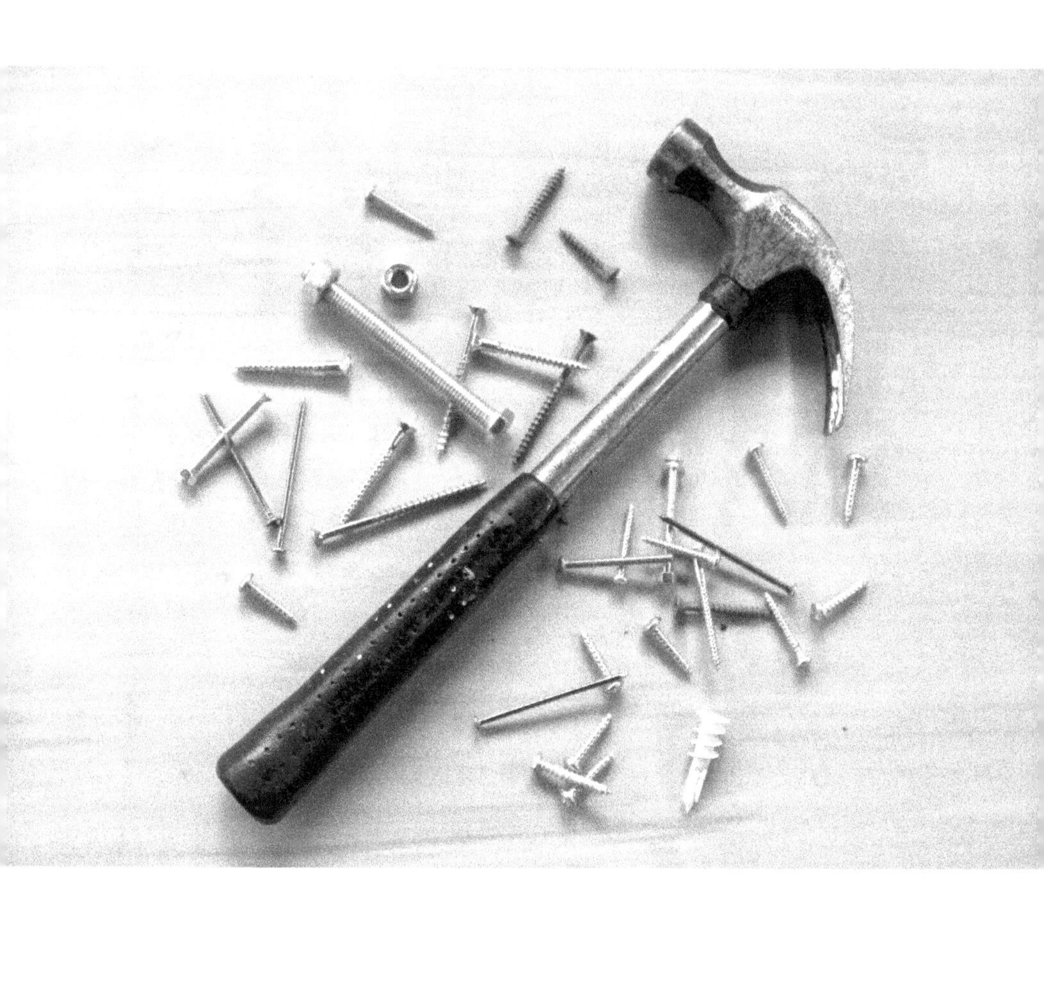

INTRODUCTION TO SCALING FORCE

All conflicts are not created equal. Sometimes your life is on the line, while other times it's just your ego. You might be able to choose whether or not to get involved, or you may find yourself with no option but to fight. The perfect response to one situation could easily prove disastrous in another. Win or lose, however, when things get physical, there will be consequences. Those consequences can be life-altering.

Some violence can be staved off simply by presence, that is, looking and acting like you're more trouble than you're worth. Bad guys don't want to fight; they want to win. And they rarely mess with alert, prepared targets. You can use words to defuse many situations, or apply calming or directive touch to reach resolution without injury. But not always. Sometimes empty-hand restraint is required, particularly if you need to control a situation without seriously hurting anyone; bouncers, security guards, and law enforcement officers routinely use such techniques. Other times, less-lethal or even lethal force is necessary to save your life or that of a loved one.

These choices form a continuum, a set of options that may be drawn upon to resolve any situation you encounter:

1. **Presence**—use of techniques designed to stave off violence via posture or body language that warns adversaries of your readiness and ability to act or that poses no threat to another's ego.
2. **Voice**—use of techniques designed to verbally de-escalate conflict before physical methods become necessary.
3. **Touch**—use of techniques designed to defuse impending violence or gain compliance via calming or directive touch.
4. **Empty-hand restraint**—use of techniques designed to control an aggressor through pain, or force compliance through leverage.

5. **Less-lethal force**—use of techniques or implements designed to incapacitate an aggressor while minimizing the likelihood of fatality or permanent injury.
6. **Lethal force**—use of techniques or implements likely to cause death or permanent injury.

It's very important to enter this force scale at the right level. If you use too much or too little force, you are in for a world of hurt. Consequently, it is vital to understand the various options, knowing how and when to apply them judiciously.

It was May of 2004 when 29-year-old Jose de Jesus brought an eight-inch butcher knife to Herald Square in Manhattan, a popular tourist spot. A guy with a long history of severe mental problems, he had violently assaulted others, including relatives, before. Nearly killed one. And he planned to do so again.

Without warning, he pulled out the knife, randomly attacked 21-year-old Dmitri Malaeyeva, stabbing him in the chest. As his first victim fell, trying desperately to stem the bleeding while drawing a tortured breath through his punctured lung, de Jesus turned on another passerby and plunged the knife into his flesh.

Screaming in terror, most bystanders began running from the scene. Some dialed 911 on their cell phones. But George Robbins, a 34-year-old graphic artist, could not stand by watching the mayhem and do nothing. So he ran toward the madman, hoping to thwart his attack. Weaponless, his heroic attempt failed, and he became de Jesus' next victim.

As Robbins fell to the ground hemorrhaging, Harold Getter rushed in and tried to disarm de Jesus. The 49-year-old security guard was unarmed and his martial skills were no match for the maniac and his knife. In moments Getter also became a victim.

And then an NYPD officer arrived.

Working with a squad assigned to thwart shoplifters in Herald Square, Officer Mary Beth Diaz was in the area, heard the screams, and rushed toward the scene. She was 23-years-old, just five months out of the Academy.

"Police!" she screamed.

De Jesus turned to face her and began stalking forward brandishing his knife.

Officer Diaz drew her duty weapon, a 9MM handgun. "Drop the knife," she shouted. When he kept coming she repeated it again. "Drop the knife! Drop the knife!"

He was only ten feet away when she opened fire. Her single shot entered de Jesus' lower abdomen and smashed into his hip, shattering the bone. He screamed, doubled over, and collapsed to the ground. He continued to writhe and shriek as she disarmed and handcuffed him, ending the carnage.

De Jesus and his four victims were rushed to Bellevue Hospital, where miraculously, no one died, not even the perpetrator. Malaeyeva, who had the most grievous injuries, was listed in fair condition by his doctors later that evening. De Jesus was also listed in fair condition after surgery. He told detectives that he had wanted to die and was hoping to goad a police officer into killing him by randomly stabbing and slashing people.

Officer Diaz was consoled by other officers and treated for trauma at the hospital. Afterward she told a reporter, "Thank God the guy is alive. Thank God I stopped him before he hurt someone else."

If you try to use Level 4 in a Level 5 situation, you will get hurt. Perhaps badly. If you try to use Level 5 in a Level 4 situation, on the other hand, you will likely wind up in jail. Or be sued. Or both. We are not just talking legalities here; you have to be able to live with yourself afterward too.

Martial artists learn dangerous, even deadly techniques. Classical systems were developed long before the advent of modern medicine. In those days, any injury sustained from a fight could be catastrophic. A busted jaw, or even a few lost teeth, might mean you'd starve to death. In the days before social services, a broken arm or leg boded poorly for your long-term chances of survival when you could no longer work for your living. Internal bleeding, a ruptured organ, or a severe concussion; forget about it—you almost certainly would not have survived.

Knowing that the shorter the fight, the lower the chance of debilitating injury, the ancient masters built systems designed to stop adversaries as quickly and ruthlessly as possible. The modern rule-of-law concept and associated legal repercussions had not been invented yet. This put 'em down, take 'em out mentality worked great at the time. If it didn't work, the styles would not still be around today. Those tactics and techniques worked so well that contemporary systems often have foundations built upon traditional methods.

The challenge is that the very same applications that may have kept you safe in the feudal times have limited utility today. It is not that they don't work, but rather that they work so well that they can only be used in certain circumstances. The brutal beat-down you deliver on the other guy might well save your life, but in the wrong circumstances, it will also land you in jail. For a really long time. Or it might make your opponent and his lawyers wealthy at your expense. Conversely, if you take the beat-down yourself, you could be seriously injured, permanently disabled, or killed.

That is why scaling force is so important. It is holistic and style-agnostic. Most importantly, it works in any situation to ensure that you will choose the right level of force when you need to use what you have learned in the *dojo* to defend yourself on the street.

For years, police agencies have used different versions of a force continuum to teach rookies how to judiciously choose an appropriate level of force, as well as to educate citizens and juries in what constitutes an appropriate force decision. Recently, there has been a movement away from teaching in this manner. The most commonly quoted reason is that officers and juries will see the continuum as a game of "connect the dots" where each level must be tried before escalating to the next. It has never been taught this way and we know of no case where an officer or a jury explained a bad decision in this manner.

The more compelling reason for many agencies abandoning an official force continuum is that the courts do not use it to adjudicate cases. Since Graham v. Connor 490 U.S. 386 (1989), it has been recognized that "the calculus of reasonableness must embody allowance for the fact that police officers are often forced to make split-second judgments—in circumstances that are tense, uncertain, and rapidly evolving—about the amount of force that is necessary in a particular situation." To many, it appears that this is exactly what codifying a force continuum is attempting to do.

Remember this: You do not work under a departmental use of force policy. You may, however, need to act in self-defense and you must act within the law. The levels of force described in this book are not prescriptive. We will not tell you, "If you are facing X, then response level Y is appropriate." That is, and will always be, the call of the person on the ground.

In Graham v. Connor, the Supreme Court stated: "The reasonableness of a particular use of force must be judged from the perspective of a reasonable officer on the scene, rather than with the 20/20 vision of hindsight. Not every push or shove, even if it may later seem unnecessary in the peace of a judge's chambers, violates the Fourth Amendment." This logic can be applied to civilian cases and criminal prosecutions as well.

There are six levels of force described in this book. While you may never need to use all of them, what we will say to you, and what we expressly believe, is that if your training does not cover the full range of skills presented here, there are situations in which you will have no appropriate options. More often than not, that will end badly.

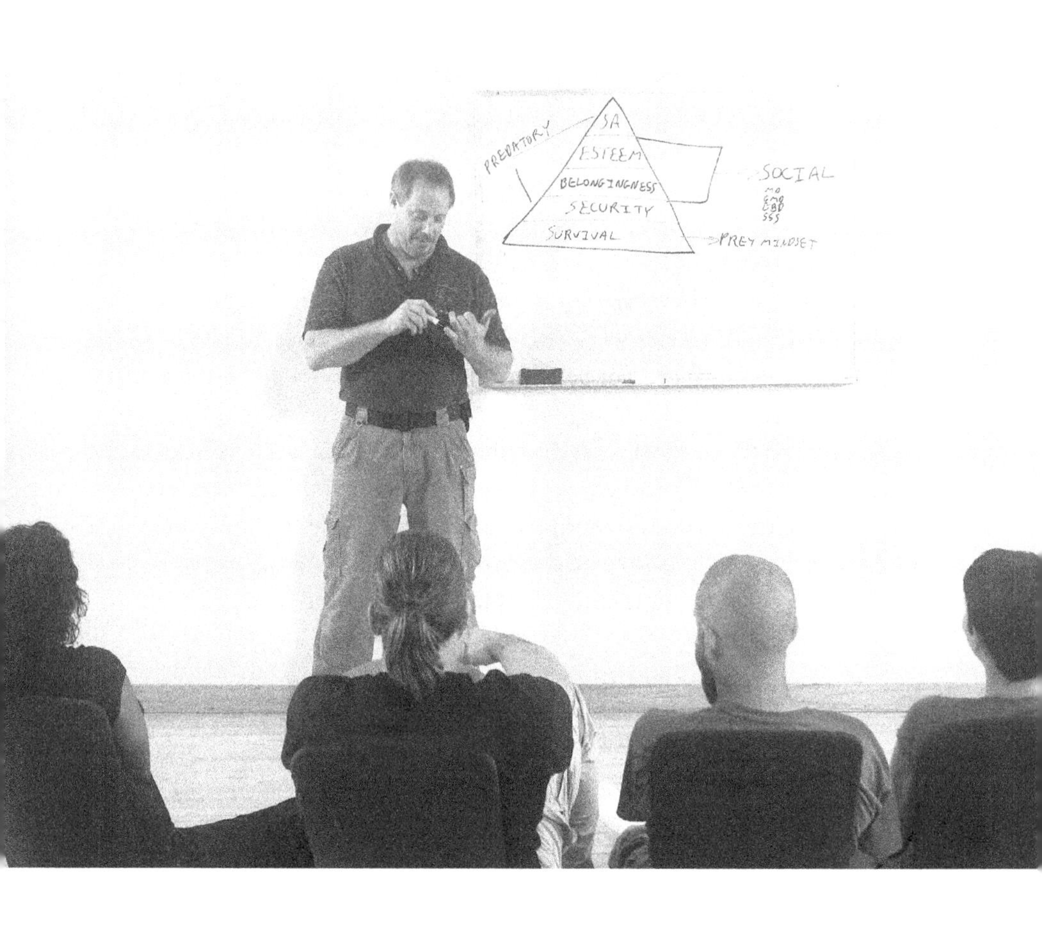
PREDATORY
SA
ESTEEM
BELONGINGNESS
SECURITY
SURVIVAL
SOCIAL
PREY MINDSET

PREREQUISITES

Even if you have never completed a woodworking project, you probably know that you *could* pound nails with a drill. You also know that it's not a horribly effective method of doing it. And it is really tough on the drill. If you want to drive nails, then a hammer is a much better choice. Clearly, knowing your tools makes any woodworking project go more smoothly.

Similarly, a scale of force options gives you a set of tools for managing violence. It also provides a basis for selecting the appropriate application to use in any given situation. The first three levels—presence, voice, and touch—can help stave off violence before it begins, precluding the need to fight. The last three levels—empty-hand restraint/physical control, less-lethal force, and lethal force—are applied once the confrontation becomes physical. Choosing the right level of force lets you control a bad situation in an appropriate and effective way, increasing your chances of surviving without serious injury while simultaneously reducing the likelihood of adverse consequences from overreacting or under-reacting, such as jail time, debilitating injury, or death.

Before you can choose the proper tool, however, it is important to understand the environment in which you will use it. That's what this section is about. If you have read our other books, much of this material will be familiar to you. Yet it bears repeating because the sections lay out important fundamentals that you need to keep in mind. Our intent is not to go in-depth, but rather to present an overview that places the various force options into the proper context.

Introduction to Violence

I'd thrown...ahem...escorted more than twenty people out of the stadium that day, but I recognized him anyway. Sometime during the third quarter, he'd taunted a Coug fan one too many times and gotten a nice shiner on his left eye for it. But the cops assigned to help us manage the end zone were busy dealing with another altercation, so I gave him the option of leaving of his own volition. When I explained what he faced in terms of minor in possession, drunk in public, disorderly conduct, and assault, he made the wise choice and voluntarily missed the rest of the game. I confiscated his ticket, marched him out the gate, and summarily forgot about him.

But he hadn't forgotten about me.

Nearly two hours later after the contest had finished and we'd gotten the stadium cleared, I spotted him in the parking lot. Not the public lot where tailgaters were still partying, but the credentialed employee parking lot where he did not belong. Unfortunately he recognized me too.

"You're the SOB who threw me out," he spat. Well it was a bit more colorful than that, but you get the idea…

Then he lunged.

Holy fuck, there's a knife in his hand! I'm still in uniform, but totally alone. No backup, no radio. My mind is spinning, but my body reacts without conscious thought. I'd been practicing saifa kata for the last few months, so that's my instinctive response.

I set a fence with my left arm, pivoting to the side. He's still drunk. And slow. Nevertheless, the knife looks like a freaking sword as it flashes by. Checking his knife-hand arm with my shoulder, I smash him in the face with a left palm-heel. His head snaps back, but he starts to retract his hand for another strike. I grab his forearm, place my right elbow on his upper arm, and drop my weight. He loses balance, dropping with me and his head smashes into the back of my fist with a thwack. As his eyes un-focus, I'm able to grab the knife and spin away, wrenching it from his grasp.

Eyes big as saucers, he twists away, stumbles once, nearly falls, then runs off. I look down at the knife in my hand.

Shit, there's blood all over me!

I start shaking so hard it slips from my grip, nearly skewering my foot when it clatters to the pavement. Heartbeat pounding in my ears, I bent over to pick it up. Bile rises, puke splashing atop the knife and my boot. Ugh, I abandon the mess, race to my car, and grab a water bottle.

I can't entirely wash away the mess, but at least the acrid taste is no longer in my mouth. I scrub my left hand clean, searching for the wound. Nothing. The blood was his.

Most martial artist's "experience" with fighting stems from sparring, tournament competitions, or the occasional schoolyard brawl. For most everyone else, it comes from Hollywood movies, televised sporting events. You may think you understand what you are participating in, or know what you are seeing, yet the realities of violence are not what most people think. In essence, there are two types of violence, social and predatory. In the former, you are fighting over a matter of face or status, while in the latter you may be fighting for your life.

The intent when it comes to blows in a social violence situation is to affect your environment. In other words, you want to establish dominance, to "educate" somebody, to get him out of your territory or something similar. There are virtually always witnesses, because you are seeking status from the outcome, either by beating the other guy down or by making him back off. Predatory violence, on the other hand, is a whole different beast from social disputes. There are usually no witnesses unless the predator has screwed up (or they are his accomplices). While the pickpocket might operate in a crowd, the mugger, serial killer, repeat rapist, arsonist, etc., generally won't.

It is relatively easy to de-escalate impending social violence so that things won't get physical, particularly if you are willing to lose face. Clever words are more important in these encounters. Unfortunately, the very factors that might de-escalate a social situation will almost certainly trigger a predatory attack if they make you appear weak. It's only possible to de-escalate predatory violence by appearing to be too dangerous to attack. If you're alert, aware, prepared, in decent physical condition, and capable of setting a verbal boundary, those are all major warning signs to the predator. Most will subconsciously pick up the fact that you have martial arts training simply by the way you stand and breathe during the confrontation. We'll delve into this difference later in more detail.

Social violence can be a big deal, predatory violence even more so; these are situations where you may be forced to defend yourself. Sparring, tournament competitions, and the like are often called "fights" by their promoters, yet these events have virtually nothing to do with fighting. To begin, fighting is illegal. Sure, you may be able to get away with it using a legitimate claim of self-defense, but there are no winners, trophies, or status points in a real fight. Fighting always has consequences.

Fighting versus Sport

The Raiders fan had biceps that could put Hulk Hogan to shame, and a physique that was nothing short of awesome. He stood out in a bar full of average guys, not only because he was ripped, but also because he was the only person cheering for the other team. The only one doing it vociferously anyway. For most of the first quarter and part of the second, Seahawks fans bantered good-naturedly with him, but as the home team struggled, chatter turned to insult that in turn became vitriolic.

I didn't hear what set him off, but suddenly a Seahawks fan stood up and hurled a half-full beer bottle at Raider, who kicked his table aside and charged his assailant. Ducking a wild punch, he scooped Seahawk's legs, planted his shoulder into the other guy's gut, and drove forward. It was a sweet takedown; Raider clearly had some type of martial arts experience. In seconds, they crashed to the ground with Raider on top. Sitting astride his stunned adversary, Raider threw a flurry of blows into the smaller guy's face. He seemed to be enjoying himself, right up to the point where one of Seahawk's friends kicked him in the head. Moments later, he was curled on the ground in a fetal position as half a dozen Seahawk fans put the boots to him.

It was a sports bar with no bouncers and no one to break things up, so the beat-down continued for several minutes before some of us began calling out that Raider had had enough. When they finally let off, he lay eerily still. Several minutes later, when the paramedics strapped him onto a backboard and wheeled him out to the waiting ambulance, he still hadn't moved.

The cops spent most of the second half of the game taking statements and making arrests.

Every mixed martial arts (MMA) competition or sparring tournament out there pales in comparison to the speed, ferocity, and brutality of a real fight. Sure, competitors train hard, achieve awesome levels of fitness, and become highly skilled at what they do. They risk injury in the ring too, but Olympic events such as judo or taekwondo, and MMA matches such as Ultimate Fighting Championship (UFC) or Pride Fighting are first and foremost sporting events. If they were not, many competitors would not survive the competition. And promoters would wind up in jail. Or get sued out of business.

These contests have rules that either ban techniques outright or change the way they are applied. In judo, for example, you pin an opponent face up so that he has a sporting chance to break your hold. Yet in the *koryu* jujutsu from which it originated, practitioners were taught to pin face down in the same way that modern law enforcement officers do for handcuffing. Done properly, the adversary cannot continue to fight that way unless he is significantly stronger than you or another person intervenes on his behalf. Furthermore, applications that are especially effective on the street, particularly if you are a smaller or weaker combatant, are not allowed because they are far too dangerous in the ring. Take the UFC for example; they outlaw the following:

- Head-butts
- Eye gouges
- Throat strikes
- Grabbing the trachea
- Biting
- Hair pulling
- Groin striking
- Fishhooking
- Putting your finger into any orifice or into any cut or laceration on an opponent

- Small-joint manipulation
- Striking to the spine
- Striking the back of the head
- Striking downward with the point of your elbow
- Clawing, pinching, or twisting the opponent's flesh
- Grabbing the clavicle
- Kicking the head of a grounded opponent
- Kneeing the head of a grounded opponent
- Stomping a grounded opponent
- Kicking the other guy's kidney with your heel
- Spiking an opponent to the canvas so that he lands on his head or neck
- Throwing an opponent out of the ring
- Holding the shorts or gloves of an opponent
- Spitting at an opponent
- Engaging in an "unsportsmanlike" conduct that causes an injury to an opponent
- Holding the ropes or the fence
- Using abusive language in the ring or fenced area
- Attacking an opponent during a break period
- Attacking an opponent who is under the care of the referee
- Attacking an opponent after the bell has sounded the end of a period
- Disregarding the referee's instructions
- Interference by someone in the competitor's corner

Recognize anything that might be useful in a street fight on that list? If you're assaulted by a larger, stronger adversary, then eye gouges, throat strikes, and the like may be exactly the right techniques to use in order to save your life. But they are too dangerous for the ring. These rules are designed not only to prevent serious injuries but also to give competitors a sporting chance to succeed. In order to keep things moving (and more interesting for the audience), the UFC takes points away from a competitor for "timidity," including avoiding contact with an opponent, intentionally or consistently dropping the mouthpiece, or faking an injury. Unlike the bar fight during the Seahawks game, they also require that competitors challenge each other one at a time.

Then there is protective gear. UFC competitors are required to use padded gloves, mouth-guards, and groin protection. In some sports, chest-guards, headgear, and other equipment is required as well.

Sporting competitions have weight classes too. Under UFC rules, competitors are grouped into lightweight (over 145 pounds to 155 pounds), welterweight (over 155 to 170 pounds), middleweight (over 170 to 185 pounds), light heavyweight (over 185 to 205 pounds), and heavyweight (over 205 to 265 pounds) divisions. Because bad guys rarely pick fights they don't expect to win, you are likely to be attacked by someone much larger or stronger on the street than you would be in the ring.

On the street, fights rarely last more than a few seconds, but when they do, there is no stopping until it's done, someone intercedes, or the authorities arrive to break things up. This is very different from sporting competitions where there are set time periods. UFC non-championship bouts run three, five-minute rounds, for example, whereas championship matches last five rounds. There is a one-minute rest period between rounds. If combatants take a break during a street fight, there's something very strange going on.

In the ring, you can win by submission (tap or verbal), knockout, technical knockout, decision, disqualification, or forfeiture. On the street, you "win" by surviving. That is quite a difference. Don't confuse sports with combat or misconstrue entertainment with reality. Fighting is ugly. It has few, if any, rules beyond the laws of physics and many serious repercussions. Sport is entertainment.

Social Violence

"You want to take it out on the ice kid? We can go right now. I'll fuck you up!" This was a 40-something- year-old guy snarling at a couple of 13-year-olds at a hockey game. The Thunderbirds had just scored a goal and the kids were celebrating along with the rest of the home crowd. This guy, a Winterhawks fan, looked like he was about to take a swing at them.

"What's going on," I asked.

"You've got to control your fucking kids. He does that again I'm gonna fucking take him out!"

"What, you're threatening a little kid. Really?" That was aimed more at his wife than him. She pretended not to notice. Others seated nearby got the message though.

"Damn right I am!"

"What did he do to piss you off man?"

"He was screaming, clapping in my fucking face."

"Did he touch you?"

"Huh?"

"Did he touch you?" I de-cloaked a little: weight shift, deadeye stare, slight edge to my voice.

"No." He quickly turned away, pretending to be engrossed in the game.

Sure, the "oh shit I killed him" thing can occur, so all violence needs to be taken seriously, but the intent in a social violence situation is to affect your environment. In other words, you want to establish dominance, to "educate" somebody, or to get him out of your territory. Sometimes that goal can be accomplished verbally, or whereas other times physical actions are necessary. Either way, social violence usually comes with instructions on how to avoid it. For example, if the other guy says, "get the fuck out of my face," he has told you exactly what will prevent escalation to violence…

One key to social violence is the presence of witnesses, people who the adversary is playing to. He may be trying to establish status, deliver an educational beat-down, or even gang together with his friends to stake out territory. In most cases, however, there is an audience of his same social class to observe his actions. If he is going to win, he will want someone around to see it. Conversely, if he is at risk to lose, the presence of others may give him a way out that won't adversely impact his reputation.

Social violence can be roughly broken into the following categories:

- The Monkey Dance
- The Group Monkey Dance

- The Educational Beat-Down
- The Status-Seeking Show
- The Territorial Defense

The Monkey Dance

Animals in the wild have ritualized combat between males to safely establish dominance without the likelihood of crippling injury or death. Just because it's not inherently life-threatening does not mean that accidents never occur, but the intent of the altercation is not to kill the opponent. Similarly, humans frequently delineate their social positions through fistfights and other unarmed conflict.

Most people who frequent bars or nightclubs have seen the glaring, staring, sizing-each-other-up type of conflicts, many of which start with the ubiquitous "what are you looking at" game. In many cases, there is an expectation that others will break up the fight or otherwise give a face-saving way out once status has been established.

Monkey dances are almost always initiated with someone whom the aggressor sees as close to his social level. (Although females occasionally exhibit similar behaviors, this is predominantly a male thing.) There is no status to be gained by a grown adult monkey-dancing with a child or elderly person. Similarly, regular people will not attempt to monkey dance with a very high-ranking individual. Mid-level people in everything from biker gangs to corporate management constantly jockey for position, but they do not do it with the folks in charge. It's too much of a leap. Challenging the group's senior leaders like that tends to be career limiting, to say the least.

The Group Monkey Dance

The group monkey dance is about solidarity, aimed at discouraging outsiders from interfering with the group's business or as a way to establish territory. Sometimes the victim is an insider who betrayed the group or stepped way out of line. In these cases, the fight can become a contest of showing loyalty to the group by determining who can dish out the most damage to the victim, a horrific and dangerous thing that rarely ends well. Unlike an individual monkey dance, the group monkey dance can easily end with a murder, even when killing the victim was not the goal.

The Educational Beat-Down

In some places or elements of society, if you do something rude and inconsiderate, you could be socially excluded or ostracized. In others, you will have the tar beaten out of you for your indiscretion. It's sort of a spanking between adults, an extreme show of displeasure designed to enforce the "rules."

If the recipient did not do something horrific to initiate the attack and properly acknowledges the wrong, an educational beat-down can be over quickly and end without significant or lasting injury. Not understanding or conceding the wrongdoing or repeated behavior that is outside the group's rules, on the other hand, can lead to a beat-down designed to maim or kill the victim.

The Status-Seeking Show

In certain segments of society, such as criminal subculture, a reputation for violence can be very valuable. This reputation can lead others to treat you more respectfully for fear of your "going off" on them. The challenge is that for someone to be truly feared and respected, they may feel a need to do something crazy beyond the bounds of "normal" social violence, such as attacking a child, disabled individual, law enforcement officer, or elderly person. It's still social violence because it is designed to develop status for the aggressor, yet the outcome could easily be fatal for the victim.

The Territorial Defense

Defending one's territory against "other" members of different social groups is fairly common in certain aspects of society such as gang culture. It's an "us versus them" worldview with violence aimed at people who look, act, or dress differently than the group. The act may be as benign as driving someone out of the group's territory or as malevolent as shooting a person for straying onto a gang's turf. Territorial defense is a bridge between social and asocial violence because while it is a defense of the group's turf or resources, it is often carried out in a manner that is profoundly asocial. This type of conflict is deliberately developed and maintained by the leaders of the involved group.

Predatory Violence

> Venkata Cattamanchi thought he was about to get lucky. He was dead wrong. He'd met a woman online who agreed to meet him for a tryst at the EZ Rest Motel in Southfield, Michigan (near Detroit). He was surprised to discover not one, but two women in the room upon arrival, yet the romantic encounter abruptly took a sinister turn when two men showed up as well. Things went downhill from there...
>
> Kevin Huffman, 28, and James Randle, 35, were convicted of ambushing, robbing, and killing Cattamanchi, in part due to statements by the two women who pled guilty to second-degree murder in exchange for their testimony. Huffman and Randle face life in prison for premeditated murder.

Predatory violence is a whole different beast from social disputes. Violence is either a means to an end or, in the case of process predators, it is the goal itself. Or it might be somebody who wants to do really bad things to you simply because he can. Predators are usually solitary because it is hard for antisocial people to band together for common purpose for any length of time. There are generally no witnesses to the attack, or the person is playing to someone of a different social class where his actions make no logical sense. For example, an adult playing the "what are you looking at" game with a child or elderly person is not going to gain any status from the outcome, whatever it may be.

There are two basic types of predators: resource and process.

Resource predators

A resource predator wants something badly enough to take it from his victim by force. Examples include muggers, robbers, or carjackers. Such aggressors are often armed. If intimidation alone works, the resource predator may not hurt you, such as in a carjacking scenario where if the vehicle is surrendered quickly, the victim is almost always left behind uninjured. A ten-year Bureau of Justice Statistics study showed that while 74 percent of all carjackings were perpetrated by armed individuals, only 0.004 percent led to murder. Because auto-related abductions were thrown into the mix, the homicide rate from carjackings could potentially be even lower than that.

Process predators

Process predators, on the other hand, act out in violent ways for the sake of the violent act itself. They are extraordinarily dangerous. Unless the process predator perceives that you are too costly to attack, it's going to get physical. You do not have to win, but you absolutely cannot afford to lose. The situation needs to end immediately. It may require you take a human life to come out as intact as possible. Rapists and serial killers are examples of process predators. A fight with a process predator frequently ends with someone in the hospital or morgue.

Situational Awareness

When we came on shift, Day Shift passed on that four of the inmates assigned to the kitchen had refused to go to work. That's odd by itself. Working can cut serious time off a sentence. Refusing to work is automatic "hole time"—a trip to disciplinary segregation. Kitchen jobs were considered a good deal and were in high demand with inmates. Odd.

An hour or so into the shift, some inmates on the kitchen crew were caught stealing cookies. That's not uncommon. Big surprise, but most people who get to jail don't have a lot of ethical hang-ups about stealing. What was surprising was that they almost wanted to be caught.

Still, it wasn't my area. Another sergeant had the East End. I was dealing with the Mental Health units on the West End.

Then a backup call. When the officer tried to cut the cookie-thieves some slack and NOT send them to segregation, they refused. They wanted to go to the hole.

This was bad. If you don't work in the system, you might not see it right away, but situational awareness is all about the situation. A jail or prison kitchen is like any other industrial kitchen. It contains a lot of things that can double as improvised weapons—knives, steam cauldrons, pots, pans, and the like. This one had 20 inmates, four civilian cooks to supervise them, and a single, unarmed officer assigned to maintain control.

Something was going to happen and whatever it was, it was so bad almost half of the inmates wanted no part of it. They were willing to go to the hole and even do extra time to not be in that kitchen on that day.

I called Lt. Turney. "This could be bad, sir. No way to be sure but it smells like a build-up to a potential hostage situation."

"I can spare you one officer. Do what you can."

"Can I have Craig?"

"Sure."

Craig was a former Marine, one of my CERT members and a thoroughly good man in a crisis. I knew and trusted his ability in a fight. More importantly, I trusted his judgment, common sense, and people skills. What we were about to do was all people skills.

Just adding two unarmed officers to the mix didn't change the odds that much. If things went bad we would still be heavily outnumbered and out-armed. But we weren't there to fight. For the next few hours, Craig and I were everywhere. Talking, listening, and telling jokes.

Nothing happened. I'll never know if something was really going to happen. But I wouldn't bet against it. And if I'm right, we changed that. Sometimes nothing is the perfect outcome.

Most self-defense experts agree that for the average citizen, the majority of dangers can be identified and avoided simply by learning how to look out for them. If you do things right, it is possible to talk your way out of more than half of the potentially violent situations that you cannot avoid. Together, this strategy means that you should only need to fight your way out of three, four, or at worst, five of every hundred hazardous encounters. With good situational awareness, you may not have anywhere near a hundred such confrontations in your lifetime so those odds really aren't all that bad.

So what is situational awareness? At the simplest level, it is knowing what is going on around you. More specifically, it is the ability to identify, process, and comprehend factors that can be important for your safety and welfare, such as the existence of potential threats, escape routes, and weapons.

Can you remember a time when you were driving along the highway, suddenly "knew" the car beside you was going to swerve into your lane, and took evasive action to avoid an accident? Almost everyone who drives has done that on numerous occasions. It is so common that most of us forget about such incidents shortly afterward. This ability to predict what other drivers are going to do is an excellent example of good situational awareness. If you fail to pay attention to what is going on around you, fixate on one task, or become preoccupied with work or personal matters, you can lose the ability to detect important information that can place you in danger when you are in a public place. In the driving example, talking or texting on your cell phone may diminish your ability to detect another driver about to move into your lane. Distracted driving causes a lot of accidents.

Knowing when it is time to leave a party is another example of good situational awareness. Fights at parties tend to happen after a certain time of night. It's not the hour on the clock that is important, but rather the mood of the crowd. Most people have a good time and leave long before the fecal matter hits the oscillating blades. Just about everyone who is going to hook up has already done so; they've found a date, left together, and are off having fun. As the crowd starts to thin, those who have nothing better to do than cause trouble are the ones who are left. Buzzing with frustration and raging hormones, those who insist on hanging on well into the night are the ones who get caught up in it when the shit is most likely to fly. If you pay attention to the behaviors of those around you, however, it's fairly easy to know when it is time to leave. If you are not there when things start to get rough, bad things cannot happen to you.

The same dynamics happen in just about any location or situation. By surveying and evaluating your environment, you achieve more control over what happens to you. Good situational awareness helps you make yourself a hard target by eliminating easy opportunities for those who wish to do you harm. It is not a guarantee of safety because there are no absolutes when it comes to self-defense, yet good situational awareness can let you predict and avoid most difficult situations.

Situational awareness, in general, is a skill that everyone instinctively has, yet few individuals pay attention to it. In most cases, you should be able to spot a developing situation and leave before anything bad happens. Pay attention to your built-in survival mechanisms, your gut feelings if you will. Once you begin to do this habitually, you will dramatically improve your safety. Your awareness skills can also be refined and improved through practice in much the same way that predicting other drivers' behavior becomes easier over time.

Sometimes, however, try as you might to avoid it, trouble finds you and you must react accordingly. Good awareness helps you be prepared for that as well. It can be used before, during, and after a fight.

No one can maintain an elevated level of awareness at all times in all places. There is a difference between being aware and becoming paranoid. Any time you are near others, however, especially strangers, it pays to be vigilant so as not to be caught unawares by sudden conflict. This simply means looking for and paying attention to anything that stands out from the norm, not only things that you see, smell, or hear, or in some cases touch, but also other's reactions to things that you cannot detect directly.

You cannot walk around in a constant state of hypervigilance, however. It's emotionally and physically untenable. Consequently, it is important to scale your awareness up or down depending on whatever you encounter around you.

Low-level awareness is essential any time you are out in public. You should be able to identify, without looking twice, generally who and what is around you. Know about vehicles, people, building entrances, street corners, and areas that might provide concealment for a threat or a source of cover to escape toward should something untoward happen.

Be self-assured and appear confident in everything you do without presenting an overt challenge or threat to others. Predators typically stalk those they consider weaker prey, rarely victimizing the strong. We are not just talking about hardcore criminals here, but also bullies and petty thugs as well. Walk with your head upright, casually scanning your immediate area as well as what is just beyond. See who and what is ahead of you, be aware of the environment to each side, and occasionally turn to scan behind you as you move.

If you become aware of some nebulous danger, something out of place, pay attention to it, but not to the exclusion of a broader awareness of your surroundings. Trouble may be starting in other places in addition to the one that has drawn your attention (for example, an ambush situation). You may have heard a nearby shout, the sound of glass breaking, or an unidentified sudden noise where you would not have expected one. You might also have seen another person or a group of people acting abnormally, someone whose demeanor makes you feel uncomfortable, somebody whose appearance or behavior stands out as unusual, or a group who appears to be reacting to something you cannot see.

Higher-level awareness is appropriate if the threat you identify appears to be aimed at you. That is where you may need to verbally de-escalate or physically control a situation. You will need to be aware of bystanders who may be potential threats or sources of aid, escape paths, impromptu weapons, and other factors depending on the tactical situation you find yourself in.

To practice situational awareness, try watching a crowd at a mall, nightclub, or other public area. Pretend that you are a bad guy and think about who you would choose as your "victim" and consider why you think that way. Who looks like a victim and who does not? What about their posture makes them appear to be a target of opportunity. How do they move? Are they paying attention to what is going on around them? Are their hands in their pockets or encumbered by packages, or are they held loosely in front of them? Are they armed? Where do their eyes move and what do they focus on? Who notices you watching? How do they react?

The victim interview

I was parked alongside a major street in downtown Seattle. My hands were full of boxes and the mid-afternoon sun was glaring in my face, making it hard to see despite my polarized glasses, so it took a couple tries to get my key into the lock. I awkwardly dragged the door open, nearly dropping some of my packages, and began shoving my purchases in to the car.

If he hadn't spoken, I wouldn't have known he was there. "Hey buddy, you know what time it is?"

While his question seemed innocuous, the fact that he was standing a foot away from me when he asked set alarm bells ringing in my head. I hurriedly threw the last box into the vehicle, more to get it out of my hands than for anything else, shifted slightly away from the car, and spun to face him. Simultaneously, I relaxed my posture, straightened my spine, and held my hands out low between me and him.

He didn't look overly threatening despite his proximity, and his hands were empty, but he was wearing a timepiece on his right wrist. "Sorry man, I don't have a watch," I replied.

The smirk on his face disappeared as he took in my posture. Muttering something I couldn't understand over the traffic noise, he buggered off clearly looking for a less prepared victim. As he walked away, I spotted a suspicious bulge, either pistol or large knife stuffed into his waistband beneath his untucked shirt.

Criminals like to dish out pain, but they aren't so keen to be on the receiving end of it. Becoming injured in a confrontation not only diminishes their ability to make a living by preying on others, but also sets them squarely in the sights of other predators higher up the food chain. Consequently, before a bad guy tees off on you, he will evaluate his odds of success. This evaluation is often called an "interview." Unlike a job search, this is one interview that you don't want to pass.

If you are not paying attention to your environment and appear to be an easy target, you are likely to be selected as the bad guy's next victim. This interview may be conducted by a single individual or a group of thugs. It may take place quickly or you may be stalked over a period of time. Regardless, your goal in such situations is to be both calm and resolute. Don't start anything you don't have to, but be prepared to fight if necessary. While most people look at someone's size and physique, experienced predators know how to recognize a threat from a person's posture or movement.

If you are approached by a single individual, be wary of bystanders who may join him. Don't forget to glance behind you when prudent because he may have an accomplice(s). Use sound, smell, reflective surfaces, and shadows to sense what is going on where you cannot look. Furthermore, pay attention to escape routes should you need to fight your way free. Be wary of the other guy's hands, particularly if you cannot see both of them because he may very well be armed and preparing to use his weapon against you.

The less you look and act like a victim during the interview process, the safer you will be. Many self-defense instructors use "woofers" who play the bad guy's role in this process so that you can experiment safely. You learn how to deal with tense situations through scenario training where your teachers debrief your performance afterward. These drills are an excellent way to prepare for interviews on the street.

The 4 D's

We think it was Geoff Thompson who originated this concept. The 4 D's is an excellent, easy to remember way of describing dirty tricks that sneak attackers often use to disguise their intent, get close enough to launch their assault, and keep you from responding until it is too late to defend yourself. This concept is an extension of the interview process. You are singled out as a potential victim, and then the bad guy(s) uses dialogue, deception, distraction, and destruction to set you up and take you down:

- **Dialogue** creates a distraction while letting your adversary control the distance between you. It is the setup to get him close enough to his intended victim where he can use the element of surprise to strike with impunity. That means that he must be within three to five feet away in order to hit you with anything other than a projectile weapon. The closer he is, the less warning you get and the harder it is to defend yourself. A guy with a watch asking you the time is a bit more obvious than typical, but a good example of the principle nevertheless. You may be asked for directions, the time, or a cigarette. While the other guy is talking, he will be evaluating your awareness, calculating his odds of success, and stealthily positioning himself to attack.
- **Deception** disguises the predatory nature of the adversary, letting him blend into the crowd and making him appear as harmless as possible until it is too late. The idea is to assure that you will not realize that you are being threatened. Much of deception is based on body language and behavior, though it can include things like wearing clothing designed to blend in and disguise the presence of weapons too.
- **Distraction** sets up the attack, typically by asking a question or otherwise using verbal techniques. It can also include gestures or body movements such as when he suddenly widens his eyes and looks over your shoulder to get you to look behind you and expose your back.
- **Destruction** is the physical assault, robbery, rape, or murder. Or it can be something more innocuous like a picking a pocket. When violence is in the cards, if he can successfully distract you, he can get in at least one or two good blows before you realize what is going on and attempt to respond. It's very tough to fight back once you are surprised, behind the count, injured, and reeling from the pain.

Despite these 4 D's, it is exceedingly rare for the victim to be caught totally unaware. For example, even if they were sucker punched, most assault victims report that they saw the blow coming but did not have time to react. Even when long-range weapons are involved (such as firearms), fights typically begin close up. Unarmed confrontations always take place at close range once things get violent. Your level of awareness and preparedness should ratchet up a bit whenever a stranger is close enough to strike, at least until you have given him a thorough once-over and dismissed any threat.

Weapons awareness

> I was watching football when I suddenly heard sirens. I live in a quiet residential neighborhood but there is a major arterial a couple of blocks away so we tend to hear an emergency response or two from time to time. They've historically passed on by rather than stopping nearby, but this time it turns out that a man was knifed a few of blocks away. The 22-year-old victim was stabbed in the stomach, rushed to Harborview Medical Center, and listed in critical condition according to press reports. Police reported that another man drove a getaway car, but didn't give a description of the vehicle that I could find.

Unarmed individuals who tangle with weapon-wielding attackers often get hurt. Frequently quite badly. Armed assaults are far more dangerous to the victim than unarmed attacks, more than three times as likely to result in serious injury. In fact, 96 percent of the homicides in the US involve some type of weapon. These attacks are three-and-a-half times more likely than unarmed assaults to result in serious damage to the victim such as broken bones, internal injuries, loss of consciousness, or similar trauma that result in extended hospitalization. Because hand-to-hand combat against an armed assailant is often a losing proposition, it is important to learn how to spot a weapon and avoid it before it can be used against you.

With few exceptions, civilians who carry a weapon need to do so in such a way that it cannot be seen by those around them yet can be drawn in a very big hurry should the need arise. After all, you wouldn't want to be stopped every five minutes by a police officer summoned by panicked bystanders who report that you are armed. Bad guys also conceal their weapons, though more often than not to maintain the element of surprise. Either way, accessibility is key. A weapon does you no good if you cannot get to it rapidly when you need it.

Most carry techniques center on or around the waist. Law-abiding civilians who own a gun usually use a holster. Holsters make the most reliable carry systems because they rigidly affix the weapon to a specific spot on the body. That way it can always be found when it is needed, even under extreme stress. Many folding knives come with belt clips designed to hold them firmly against the side of your pocket where they are easily located by touch.

Criminals, on the other hand, rarely use a holster. The two most common ad-hoc carry positions for firearms are inside the pants, either in the front alongside the hipbone or in the small of the back. Because the weapon has a tendency to move around when carried in this fashion, you can often spot a bad guy touching himself to assure that it is in the proper place or adjusting the weapon to get it back into the proper carry position.

Pants or jacket pockets are always a handy choice as well. Like the inside-the-pants carry, they are not as reliable or easy to get to as a holster when you need rapid access. Weapons can also be palmed, hidden behind an arm or leg, or held out of sight beneath a covering object such as a folded jacket or newspaper. These methods facilitate rapid access but can be easier to spot than other methods. That's the good news. The bad news is that if the weapon is already drawn and held in a concealed position, you will be in extremely serious trouble if you do not spot your adversary's intent. He has already decided to attack and is maneuvering into position to do so.

Weapons can also be "hidden" in plain sight too. A hot cup of coffee tossed into a bad guy's face can make an effective deterrent. A solidly built pen can operate much like a martial arts *kubotan* or even like a knife. A cane, walking stick, heavy purse, or laptop computer can be used as a bludgeon. A bunch of keys on a lanyard can work much like a medieval flail, albeit far less effectively. A beer bottle, pool cue, baseball bat, or mug can be just as effective in a pinch as a weapon designed for combat.

Pay particular attention to a person's hands and midsection, looking for unusual bumps, bulges, out-of-place items of clothing, or odd movements. Also look for concealing clothing that may be covering a weapon. Examples include a jacket worn in hot weather, a vest that covers the waistline (especially the hips/lower back), or a loose shirt that is only buttoned high.

Just because a weapon is not in use at the beginning of a fight does not necessarily mean that it won't be by the end, particularly if the other guy thinks he's in danger of losing. Before, during, and even after a fight, watch for the upward or sideways motion of withdrawing a weapon from its sheath, holster, or hiding place; a weapon cannot be used until it is deployed. If someone takes one of their hands out of the fight voluntarily, it is rarely a good sign.

While you will frequently rely on your eyes to spot a concealed weapon, you can use your ears too. Listen for the sound of a weapon being drawn or readied for action as well.

Weapon awareness is relatively easy to practice. Take an outdoor seat at a restaurant in a high foot-traffic area, hang out in a mall, or take a walk through a public place, and carefully watch passersby. Count how many knives, guns, and other weapons you can spot. Who is carrying them? How are they concealed? What subtle clues did you notice that helped you spot the weapon? Once you become good at consciously finding these devices, you can begin to pick them up subconsciously as well. Honing your intuition in this manner builds solid survival skills.

Situational awareness during a fight

While the goal of situational awareness is to avoid violence in the first place, if things go south it remains an important aspect of surviving the fight. It is critical to remain aware not only of openings where you might land a blow or find an opportunity to escape but also for any changes in the dynamics of the conflict such as deployment of a weapon, intervention by third parties, hazardous terrain or obstacles, etc. This can be a challenge, particularly when adrenalized as tunnel vision is a common symptom, but it is important to pay attention to what's going on around you to the extent possible.

Sometimes an opening is nothing more than a flash of color; say a blue shirt suddenly visible behind a rapidly moving, tan forearm. Similarly a weapon might be silver or a black blur that stands out against that same shirt or the flesh of the hand that holds it. The presence of a secondary threat, such as another combatant or a moving vehicle, might be a subtle hint of movement in your peripheral vision, one that is easily ignored if you are focused solely on your adversary.

You won't always be able to see what is going on during a fight, so you need to listen too. Sounds can be vitally important. Does the crunch of a footstep mean that another person is about to join in the fray? Is the rip of Velcro pulled apart or the click of a snap being undone mean that a weapon is about to be deployed? What about calls for help, threats of intervention, or other actions by witnesses or bystanders? It's all significant.

Finally, your sense of touch is also important during a fight. For example, you may not be able to see exactly where an adversary is during a scuffle, particularly if you've got blood, sweat, or pepper spray in your eyes, but if you can grab a hold of his arm, it is a simple exercise to find his head (or other body parts) based upon that orientation. Weapons are often felt rather than seen. In a frightening example, it's extremely common for stabbing victims to think they were merely punched, yet the feel of a blade entering your flesh is different than that of a fist connecting with your body. Be aware of sensations like that too.

Blindfold sparring and slow work are great ways to gain experience finding targets by touch, but one of the best methods for increasing your situational awareness during a fight is through a one-step drill called "frisk fighting." Virtually everyone carries some type of weapon most of the time, be it a designed implement such as a knife or gun, or simply something they can use to hurt someone like a briefcase or a set of car keys.

The frisk fighting drill can be a lot of fun, but it also must be taken very seriously or someone will be hurt, maybe killed. An experienced practitioner needs to be in charge of safety. The drill can be performed in a training hall or gymnasium, but renting a nightclub or warehouse adds another level of realism. Either way, the drill area must be cordoned off, cleared of anything truly dangerous, and everyone must be checked to assure that no live weapons enter the arena or come into reach of the participants. There can be no exceptions to this.

Every drill introduces a known "flaw" to assure participant safety. In this case it's twofold, equipment and speed. Equipment first: Each participant should bring the safe training equivalent of what they carry every day. With proper equipment and oversight, this could include real firearms with Simunition®, inert pepper spray, and Shocknife™ training knives, among other tools. More often than not, however, practitioners wind up using rubber training weapons instead. Alternatively, training instruments can be strewn around the practice area where anyone can have access to them. Either way, the environment around you is as much in play as the other guy, hence the focus on safety.

Now on to speed: The drill is performed as a tandem exercise done in slow motion with each partner taking turns and multiple participants working together at the same time. This is commonly called a "one-step" training exercise. One partner initiates a move and the other partner matches his or her speed making a single motion to respond. You each get only one movement before it becomes the other person's turn. The drill continues without resetting until the allotted time expires, or you end up in a position from which you cannot continue and have to reset.

Even though you move slowly, it is vital to use proper body mechanics and targeting as well as to move at equal speed. It's okay to speed things up a bit so long as you are both doing it, in control, and safely. Keep things slow enough that you have time to evaluate and take advantage of the "best" opening available. In this fashion you are training to habituate good techniques. You can do the exact same things on the street, only faster. This drill is not about winning or losing; it's about refining your situational awareness during a fight.

Nevertheless, you should react to the opponent's blows so that the ebb and flow of the fight is more-or-less realistic. You don't need to stop moving even if you're "killed." It is important to talk to each other so that you will learn what you are doing well in addition to discovering opportunities you may have missed during the exercise.

The basic one-step drill is not so hard, but here's the twist: you can use your hands and feet along with everything else you find in the training area except what you brought into the game. If you can draw your opponent's weapon in one motion, do so, but you cannot draw your own. It's rare, but sometimes creative participants will draw a weapon from someone else in the room who is not their opponent. This kind of creativity is encouraged.

This is not a competition, but rather a cooperative endeavor, which incorporates several related skills and concepts:

- It makes people stay alert for opportunities and openings.
- It forces people who carry weapons to consider and practice weapons retention.
- It gives a (very mild) introduction to fighting in an armed world.
- It rewards an educated sense of touch—often you feel the weapon before you see it.
- It brings an elevated awareness of the environment and the people around you.

In order to truly benefit from this drill, it is critical that each person makes only one motion during their turn. Not one block and one strike but only one action. This encourages strategic movement and angles of attack, economy of motion, and techniques that simultaneously attack and defend in one movement. The habits you learn in this type of training can make a huge difference on the street where you will often be trying to recover the initiative once the threat has already attacked you.

Identifying the threat's "tell"

The Halloween crowd was rockin'. Spinnakers offered a thousand dollars for the best costume and there were over a hundred contestants. Encased in over 115 pounds of 16-gauge steel, I chatted up the "mermaid" next to me while waiting my turn to show off my outfit, a stunning replica suit of medieval white-harness plate armor. The girl was hot, but her boyfriend was hotter when he saw us laughing together. I headed over to grab a drink when he confronted me.

"Stay the fuck away from my girlfriend asshole," he spat.

"We were just talking dickhead. Get over it!"

Okay, that wasn't the smartest thing to say, but I was 22, a little drunk, and hadn't gotten over that whole raging hormone thing yet. Nevertheless, his reaction was by no means unexpected. His nostrils flared. His face turned red. He snarled. And threw a punch at my head.

Normally I'm not one to favor blocking with my face, but in that instance I just grinned at him as he broke his hand on my steel helmet. Unfortunately when the bouncers tossed him out, the girl left with him. Can't win 'em all...

While it often seems that way to victims, violence does not happen in a vacuum. There is always some type of escalation process beforehand. While it may be a long, drawn-out confrontation that builds up to the point of attack, it could just as easily appear to be a sudden ambush. In such situations, the escalation may have taken place within the mind of the aggressor. Either way, an astute observer can identify and react to cues, such as an adversary's adrenal twitch that precedes his attack. Unfortunately, if you do not spot these indicators or "tells" in common self-defense parlance, you are bound to get hurt.

Spotting an adversary's tell directly requires you to notice very small physical movements and signals of the other guy's intent to attack. These indicators are often subtle, hence easy to miss, particularly when you are distracted or mentally unfocused. For example, the tell might be a slight drop of the shoulder, a tensing of the neck, a flaring of the nostrils, or even a puckering of the lips. On the other hand, changes in an opponent's energy are much easier to spot then any specific physical sign. You are simply looking for change. Any change of energy should be treated as a danger signal. Here are some examples that you can recognize and act on during a confrontation:

- A person who was standing still moves slightly. A weight shift is far subtler than a step, but this change is a possible preparation for attack.
- There is a change in the rate, tone, pitch, or volume of a person's voice. An overt example is when someone who is shouting becomes suddenly quiet or, conversely, one who has been quiet suddenly raises his voice.
- A person who was looking at you suddenly looks away or, conversely, a person who was looking away suddenly makes eye contact. Watch this one. As humans we focus on eyes/face to gauge attention, which we think is important, but often turning the head away, especially with an experienced fighter, loads and clears the shoulders for a strike.
- There is a sudden change in the person's breathing. Untrained adversaries will begin to breathe shallow and fast in the upper chest while trained opponents will breathe slow and deep from their abdomen.
- A person develops a sudden pallor or flushing of his face (paling is adrenaline-induced vasoconstriction, reddening is vasodilation).
- There is a change in the person's posture. Untrained adversaries tend to "puff up," opening their chest and arching their spine, while trained opponents tend to close down their chest, straighten their spine, and lower their center of gravity.

These seem to be contradictory—look away or lock on, puff up or compress, pale or flush. They are not. An amateur or someone engaging in social violence is trying to send a message of domination, so they get big, red, and loud. They lock eyes so that you know who beat you. A professional tries to calm himself (abdominal breathing, slow smooth movements) and not draw attention. He looks away just before the attack to check for witnesses.

Most people aren't mentally prepared for sudden violence. Even when sucker punched, most victims see a blow coming before they are hit. But not in time to react. Those who fail to recognize the signs of an impending attack or who wait too long to take action can be needlessly hurt or killed. It does not matter why you are being attacked, simply that you are in danger. Do not deny what is happening, recognize the change of energy that constitutes your adversary's tell, and respond appropriately to defend yourself. Worry about making sense of the encounter once it is over and you are safe.

Legal Ramifications of Violence

> Recently I watched *Felon,* a movie that makes some realistic and valuable points about self-defense. The story centers around an average guy named Wade Porter (played by actor Stephen Dorff). Porter, his fiancé, and young son have just moved into their first house. After years of struggling for success, his construction business is beginning to take off, they have gotten their finances in line, the marriage ceremony is rapidly approaching, and life is good. Of course this happiness doesn't last. One night an intruder breaks into their home and everything changes. Porter hears a noise, finds a guy in his son's bedroom, chases him outside, and smacks him in the head with a baseball bat, killing him. Since the burglar was unarmed and died outside the home where castle doctrines do not apply, Porter is sentenced to three years for voluntary manslaughter.
>
> As the movie progresses, Porter soon realizes that he has lost everything over a split-second decision. The movie teaches some valuable lessons. Chasing down an unarmed intruder who's hell-bent on escaping and attacking him is clearly not self-defense, not even in Hollywood. In fact, in most jurisdictions a person can only resort to deadly force in order to escape imminent and unavoidable danger of death or grave bodily harm. That "unavoidable" part is the bugger.

Let's be honest, fighting can be fun. But there is a downside too. If you've been in a fight, there is a very good chance that you will be charged with a crime. The more damage you caused to the other guy, the more serious that crime may be. Consequently, it is important to know where and when you are legally justified in getting physical and when you are not.

Legal definitions and interpretations are not universal. To stay out of jail, you really need to talk to an attorney who understands the laws and nuances that apply wherever you might encounter a fighting situation. In general, the classic rule is that self-defense begins when deadly danger begins, ends when the danger ends, and revives again if the danger returns. A proactive-violent defense before an attack has taken place can be extremely challenging to prove legitimate self-defense in the eyes of the court. You will need to very clearly articulate your reasoning. Similarly, a killing that takes place after a crime has already been committed is tough to prove as self-defense. Chasing a burglar outside and attacking him does not end any better in real life than it did in that movie.

Affirmative Defense

You must understand that "self-defense" is an affirmative defense. What this means is that you are admitting to an action that is a crime and arguing that you should not be punished because it was justifiable under the circumstances.

This concept is paramount and bears repeating: claiming self-defense is admitting to the basic crime.

> *Scenario:* You walk into your kitchen late one night and suddenly see a flash of steel, and a knife gets buried in your chest. In an explosive miracle of training, luck, and the will to survive, you lash out with a perfect throat shot. You dial 911 but pass out from blood loss before you can answer any questions. While you are unconscious, the home invader suffocates from the trachea you crushed.

The guy is dead. You killed him. That is homicide. The charge will likely be manslaughter technically, since it is unlikely a prosecutor would try to prove that your intent was specifically to kill. Don't get hung up on the nuances, but understand clearly that if you claim self-defense you cannot deny the underlying crime. You committed homicide, but you have a really good excuse for doing it—dude was trying to kill you. The challenge is that if your self-defense plea fails, you have admitted to a crime and you will be punished for it.

An affirmative defense, therefore, shifts the burden of proof to you. The prosecution does not need to prove that someone was killed or that you did it. You did his job for him. YOU must prove that you had no choice but to react the way you did.

I.M.O.P. Principle

How do you know when it is legal to get physical with an adversary? Learn the I.M.O.P. (**I**ntent, **M**eans, **O**pportunity, and **P**reclusion) principle. All four of these criteria must be met before you have a good case for taking action. If one or more of these conditions are absent, you are on shaky legal ground.

These guidelines are not only useful, but they are also easy to remember in the heat of the moment on the street. That's because they are based on common sense. You must be in danger, or "jeopardy" in order to protect yourself from harm. Obvious, right? Danger from another human being comes from their intent, means and opportunity.

The hard part is that knowing this is not enough. The presence of intent, means, and opportunity may be sufficient for you to act in self-defense. However, their mere presence may not be enough for you to prevail in court. You must also be able to explain how you personally knew that each element was present in a way that the jury will believe.

Intent

You must be able to show that the threat (the standard cop term for a bad guy) wanted to do you harm.* You must be able to tell how you knew. Someone screaming, "I'm going to kill you!" is fairly clear, at least if his body language backs up his words. If the threat balls up his fist and draws his hand back, you can explain why you believed he

* For self-defense. Other levels of legal force, such as refusing to leave the premises after a lawful order to do so, also require I.M.O., but at a different level.

was about to hit you. If a threat suddenly reaches under his jacket, you may believe that he is going for a weapon and can explain that too.

Intent is critical. People have chances to kill you all the time. The waiter bringing you a steak knife in a restaurant has a deadly weapon and is well within range. But we do not kill the waiter, nor do waiters live in fear, because we all understand that without intent there is no threat. No justification for force. So we don't act.

This goes for the guy reaching under his jacket. This is an action that people do every day, getting out wallets, keys, and loose change. The hand reach itself is not enough. You will have to explain all the elements of that moment that indicated to you why that action showed intent. Did he continue toward you after being told to back off? Were you in an isolated area or alone at night at an ATM? Did you see, hear, or smell something that brought this everyday movement to a new level?

To be a legitimate threat, the person must have intent **and** you must be able to explain how you knew that.

Means

All the intent in the world does not matter if the threat couldn't hurt you. Most people have some means at some level—fists and boots and size. Others have weapons or indicate that they have weapons.

A two-year-old throwing a temper tantrum has some of the purest intent in the world, but he or she lacks the size, strength, and coordination to do anything severe.

The means that the actions you articulate must also match the means that were presented. People who were poorly trained in self-defense mouth the words, "I was in fear for my life," like it is a mantra or a get-out-of-jail-free card. It is a bullshit platitude. You will be expected and required to explain exactly what made you fear for your life—the intent, the means, and the opportunity. If you are claiming the threat was deadly, the means have to be deadly. A shoving match does not count.

You must be able to articulate exactly what led to your fear in a way that demonstrates it was legitimate.

Opportunity

Intent and means do not matter if the threat cannot reach you. If someone is screaming he is going to kick your ass from across the room, he may be a threat but he is not an *immediate* threat. You can't shoot him. If he has a gun, being across a room does not matter as much. You have a pretty good argument that you were in danger. Similarly, someone waving a knife at you from inside a vehicle while you are walking on the sidewalk is not an immediate threat. If he slams the accelerator and the car lurches toward you, that situation has changed significantly.

Intent, means, and opportunity are the desire, the ability, and the access to hurt you. You must be able to show all three to justify using force for self-defense.

Preclusion

Even if intent, means, and opportunity are clear, there is one other requirement (for civilians and in most states*) to satisfy. You must be able to show that you had no safe alternatives other than physical force before engaging an opponent in combat. If you can retreat without further endangering yourself**, this criterion has not been met. After all, it is impossible for the other guy to hurt you if you are not there.

These are the questions any jury will be asked and you must be able to explain: Could you have left? Could you have run? Did you in any way contribute to the situation getting out of hand? Would a reasonable person have seen a way out or seen a way that used less force?

All of these are preclusions that would have stopped the situation

* Law Enforcement Officers have a "duty to act" and can't be expected to retreat. In some states, "Stand Your Ground" laws *appear* to remove the preclusion requirement. "Castle" laws give great freedom for self-defense in the home provided the threat feloniously enters. If someone breaks into your home, a castle law essentially grants that I.M.O. are givens.

** The justifications for defending a third party are essentially the same as for defending yourself. Though you, yourself, might be able to leave safely if another potential victim would be left behind and helpless, you can articulate why you needed to engage.

from going to force. You must not only prove the threat was real and immediate, but that you had no other good options.

Clearly you should never let fear of legal repercussions keep you from defending yourself when your life is on the line, but an understanding of the law can help you make good decisions on "that day" should it ever arrive.

Reasonable force

There are no absolutes in self-defense, but your ultimate goal is to apply sufficient force to effectively control the situation and keep yourself from harm. In general, you may legally use reasonable force in defending yourself. "Reasonable force" is considered only that force reasonably necessary to repel the attacker's force.

Unfortunately, "reasonably necessary" is a vague term usually associated with what the "reasonable person" would think necessary. The so-called reasonable person is a fictitious composite of all the reasonably prudent people in a given cross section of life.

Whether the ordinary person acted reasonably will likely be judged against the reasonably prudent, similarly situated ordinary person in the appropriate geographic area. Everyone starts out at this level, but other personal attributes may heighten their required standard of care.

Whether a martial artist acted reasonably in a fight will likely be judged against the reasonably prudent practitioner of similar skill and training in that general geographic area. This test works the same way for other experts as well. For example, whether a doctor acted reasonably in medical care will be judged against the reasonably prudent doctor of similar skill, training, and specialty.

The reasonable person standard is not necessarily used in all criminal proceedings nor is it universally used in all civil proceedings. On the other hand, some standard of reasonable and right are embedded in the mind of every person, including those sitting in the jury box. The reasonable person standard will likely also be used in any civil suit (e.g., wrongful death) filed after a criminal decision.

A trained fighter is usually held to a higher standard of reasonableness than the average person in a court of law. The martial artist's training is believed to give him or her better understanding of the application and consequences of using a certain amount of force. Thus, where a less-skilled individual might be able to shoot a club-wielding attacker, it may only be reasonable in the eyes of an undereducated jury for the martial artist to use his or her hands for defense. For non-practitioners, most folk's understanding of martial arts is limited to unrealistic movie and television stunts. This is why expert witnesses are so important (and expensive).

Crimes generally revolve around the "intent" to do something bad, or the "reckless disregard" of the consequences of doing something that turned out bad in retrospect. Reasonableness also enters criminal proceedings to help resolve issues surrounding intent or reckless disregard. You can never know with certainty what someone intended yet the courts can infer what was intended from evidence and circumstances. This inference involves knowledge, skill, training, and state of mind of the participants as applied to the evidence and circumstances at hand.

Exceeding a reasonable level of force may well turn a victim into a perpetrator in the eyes of the court. Justifiable self-defense is a victim's defense to a criminal/civil charge. If one's intent were to defend his or her self, then a reasonable person would only do so using reasonable force. Using a higher level of force infers intent to needlessly harm the other. This allows the perpetrator turned "victim" to use your defensive actions against you, the victim turned perpetrator. Even if a criminal prosecutor dismisses your actions, a civil court may not do so.

Disparity of Force

Another important aspect of self-defense is disparity of force. While there is no such thing as a fair fight in most instances, legally there is often an expectation of one. Equal-force doctrines in some jurisdictions require law-abiding citizens to respond to an attack with little or no more force than that which he or she perceives is being used against him or her. In some places, the law clearly specifies that equal force must be exactly equal. The attacked can respond with no more force than that by which he or she is threatened—slap for slap, punch for punch, kick for kick, or deadly weapon for deadly weapon.

Disparity of force between unarmed combatants is measured in one of two ways. It exists if:

- The victim is being attacked by someone who is physically much stronger or younger.
- The victim is being attacked by two or more assailants of similar or equal size.

Where disparity of force exists, you may legitimately be able to exert potentially lethal force to defend yourself. However, a person cannot legally respond to an assault of slight degree with deadly force. Such overreaction will land you in serious legal trouble.

Proportional Force

In practice, you will usually want to respond to an assault with a degree of force sufficiently, but not greatly, superior to that with which you are threatened. There are two advantages to this "slightly greater" degree of force doctrine:

- It places the defender in a more secure tactical position.
- It discourages the assailant from continuing to attack and escalating into a position where lethal force is required.

Some self-defense experts throw out the phrase, "It's better to be judged by twelve than carried by six." Though the sentiment is accurate—we would rather risk prison time than a cold grave—it trivializes the problem. Never forget that if you are found guilty in a jury trial, you will be spending a whole lot of quality time in a confined environment with unpredictable, dangerous neighbors who may be less than friendly when you interact with them. You may also suffer consequences with others in the community, facing challenges from family, friends, employers, and those you wish to interact positively with on a daily basis.

While you should never let fear of legal consequences keep you from surviving a violent encounter, you must keep your wits about you at all times.

The Articulation Drill

Good people tend to make good decisions. These decisions can always be refined and the decision-making process can be improved, but usually people don't trip themselves up much in the process; they trip themselves up in the explanation.

Having justification is not enough. I.M.O.P. by itself will not get you out of trouble. Because self-defense is an affirmative defense, it falls on you to explain. You must be able to articulate exactly why you made each decision—why you needed to become involved and why you used exactly the level of force and even technique that you used.

There are two drills for this. One is simple. Go to YouTube. Watch real fights. Then pick out exactly why it was or wasn't self-defense. Look at all the times the guy who walked away could have been fine if only he had kept his mouth shut. It was clearly a mutual fight but both thought they were defending themselves. There are times when a pre-emptive strike would have been justified, and prudent, and others where such actions land the perpetrator in jail.

The second drill, the articulation exercise, requires some background.

As we mentioned in the situational awareness section, you have a finely developed intuition. All humans do. Your senses perceive and your brain processes huge amounts of information, far more information than your conscious mind can handle. Because of this we get "feelings." Hints. Little subconscious niggles.

Next time you get an intuition, a thought, or an idea, stop and explain it to yourself. The exercise is just that simple. And that difficult. When you see two people and think, "They are about to argue," take the time to figure out what triggered that intuition. Body language? What specific body language? Did the voices change? How? Louder? Higher pitched?

This articulation exercise has two benefits. The first is simply the skill at explaining a fast decision. If you ever need to defend your use of force in court, it is likely that you will have made a decision very quickly, probably faster than conscious thought. And you may have to explain that decision to a jury.

The second benefit will affect your entire life. Intuition is a larger part of your brain, of *you*, than your conscious mind will ever be. The articulation exercise makes your conscious mind and intuition work together. It develops trust between two parts of your mind. Intuition ceases to be "mere" intuition but something you learn to trust. Not only will the drill help you to make better decisions faster, it will also help you understand and explain those decisions.

The Decision to Get Involved

On September 23, 2002, at least ten people allegedly saw 18-year-old Rachel Burkheimer bound and gagged, lying on the floor of an Everett, WA garage shortly before she was taken out into the woods and murdered. None of them stopped to help. None of them even called the police. Legally, none of them had to. Many people simply will not get involved, even in cases of life or death. Are you one of them?

You need to seriously think about what you are willing to do, what you are not willing to do, and what you are willing to have done to you far before violence occurs. Such decisions cannot rationally be made during a dangerous encounter. There is a vast continuum of responses to take should you choose to intervene in a conflict—everything from moving to a safe place and dialing 911 to taking hands-on physical action. Intervention can be verbal or physical, encompassing the entire force continuum.

Spending some time thinking about when and under what circumstances you are willing to get involved is important. While scenario training can help prepare you for such decisions, when it gets down to brass tacks every situation you encounter will be different. It's no longer a philosophical exercise. You need to know exactly what you are walking into to make a wise choice.

Start by evaluating what you have encountered. If your situational awareness is good, you might have several seconds, or possibly even minutes, to do this reconnaissance before you are forced to take action. If it's poor you may have to take in the scene and make a decision in microseconds. Or it may be made for you. In whatever time you have, do your best to note combatants, witnesses, sources of improvised weapons, terrain, and other important factors so that you will know as much as possible about what you are up against.

The decision to get involved (or not) and at what level is paramount. Whatever choice you make can have lasting consequences. There is a cost in terms of physical and/or emotional well-being to taking action as well as to not taking action. Only you can decide. And you've got to live with that choice.

Fight to the Goal

When I was twelve years old, I was walking to the bus stop after judo practice one night when four older boys stopped me. They quickly began to hassle me about the gi I was wearing, spitting on me, calling me names, and threatening to "kill" me. Verbal threats soon escalated to pushing and shoving, which was clearly evolving toward more serious blows. Although I probably stood a good chance of badly injuring one or two of them, I felt that there was no way I could win a fight against four kids, all of whom were bigger, older, and most likely stronger than I was.

Swallowing my pride, I did my best to ignore their expectorating and taunting while I tried to figure out a way to escape. As soon as I saw a car approaching, I shoved the nearest antagonist out of the way, shoulder-rolled over the hood of the vehicle, and darted across the street. The driver slammed on his brakes, stopping between where I had just run and where the bullies on the sidewalk had started to follow. While they were distracted by the irate driver, I hopped over a fence, ducked down another side street, and ran away as fast as I could. In a situation where I could not win, running was the best thing to do.

Once you make the decision to fight it is important to know why. What is your goal? Are you trying to control a situation or escape from a threat? Everything hinges on this. The strategy of control or escape will drive the tactics necessary for success.

It is very hard, for example, to capture someone who is determined to get away, even when multiple adversaries are in play. If that is your goal, simply running away may be enough, particularly if you are able to move first. If in attempting to escape, you let yourself be drawn into a fight, however, it becomes self-defeating. Knocking an adversary aside so that you can run is better than squaring up to him in this instance. After all, your goal is to escape, not to beat down the other guy, win the fight, control the adversary until authorities arrive, or whatever else you can think of.

Consider intent, means, opportunity, and preclusion when determining your goals during a conflict. Many altercations these days are captured on video, be it from surveillance systems, cell-phone cameras, dash-cams, or some other source, at least when they occur in major populations centers across the United States. Even where video is not in the picture, bystanders may witness the event. If your actions don't match your statements you will be in serious trouble when you get to court, particularly when it comes to preclusion.

Know your goal and make tactical decisions that support it.

Dealing with Threats with Altered States of Consciousness

Alcohol muddles your mind so that you don't fully think things through. It also relaxes your inhibitions so that you are more likely to act out. Oftentimes it gives you a socially acceptable excuse for your behavior, or at least portions of it, compounding the effect. You want to do more and think you'll get away with it, not that you actually will, of course... According to the Bureau of Justice Statistics, about 36 percent of all criminals and 41 percent of violent offenders are intoxicated with alcohol when they commit the crimes for which they are convicted. These numbers rise even higher if you add drugs into the mix.

Drunks can be unpredictable, violent, and very difficult to corral. Tangling with one when you are sober gives you a significant advantage. When you're drunk too, it only exacerbates the situation. Either way, you need to do your best to keep a cool head.

To begin, never argue with a drunk. As the old saying goes, "Reason goes into the bottle faster than the alcohol comes out of it." If you can get away with it, just smile, nod, and say "Yes" or "No" as appropriate. Oftentimes, however, liquid courage will lead the other guy to take a swing at you. That is when you will undoubtedly be tempted to strike back.

Unfortunately, hitting a drunk doesn't work nearly as well as you might think. It is not necessarily that they don't feel pain, but rather that they do not feel it as much or as immediately as sober people do. That is an important consideration when dealing with an inebriated opponent.

Alcohol is not the only substance you might encounter that alters the mind of those who mean you ill. People who use drugs are roughly twice as likely to engage in violent behaviors as people who do not. In general, it is best to avoid tangling with anyone who is under the influence of drugs because such confrontations can become extraordinarily ugly. Leave such things to law enforcement professionals whenever possible.

For example, it can take as many as a dozen officers to restrain someone effectively in a drug-induced frenzy without accidentally killing him because less-lethal weapons such as pepper spray, Tasers® and the like, can prove ineffective in such cases. There is a good chance that many, if not all participants, will be injured in the process.

According to the Bureau of Justice Statistics, more than half of violent criminal offenders are under the influence of drugs or alcohol, or both, at the time of their offense for which they are subsequently convicted. The drugs of choice are most often marijuana, cocaine/crack, or heroine/opiates. Stimulants such as cocaine and crack are most linked to violence, although certain psychological conditions can have similar effects. (We'll discuss emotionally disturbed persons in the chapter about Level 2.) Similarly, about 30 percent of victims are intoxicated with drugs at the time they are attacked.

Pain Compliance versus Mechanical Compliance

> At the end of the National Anthem, we block the stairs above the 50-yard line to let the band exit the field and take their places in the stands. This usually takes several minutes, during which latecomers cannot take their seats. Those at the front of the line can see the kickoff and first few plays of the game, but those in back can only hear what's going on. Needless to say that makes us somewhat less than popular, yet most fans understand and wait (more or less) patiently for the band to get out of the way. Not so, no-shirt guy. Painted purple with a gold W on his chest, he shoved his way through the line and tried to push his way past the guards at the top of the stairs.
>
> They managed to stop his forward progress, but he launched into a verbal tirade and continued to push against my employees, nearly knocking one down the cement stairwell. After helping the guard regain his balance, I stepped into the fray and tried to reason with the fan, quickly discovering that he was far too intoxicated to understand what I was saying let alone comply. After fruitlessly arguing for a moment, I reached over and slid my fingers around the top of his collarbone while simultaneously pushing my thumb into the suprasternal notch at the base of his throat and dug in hard. On most people this will cause excruciating pain, simultaneously buckling their knees. On this guy, nothing. He didn't even notice.

Pain compliance is a an excellent tool. It affords you the ability to control an opponent without seriously injuring him—when it works. Unfortunately, a committed adversary, a person whose mind is affected by certain intoxicants or who is in an altered state of consciousness, or one who is gripped by adrenaline is likely to shrug off virtually any pain you can throw at him. In those cases, pressure points or pain compliance techniques will not be enough. You will need mechanical leverage to control or injure your adversary.

If you must hurt someone in a fight, you will need to target a vital area of his body, someplace that can be damaged relatively easily. Punching someone in the stomach, for example, may only piss him off while striking him in the head may render him unconscious if you hit hard enough (and possibly shatter your hand in the process).

As we cover the higher levels of the force continuum, you will discover that targeting moves from lesser to more vital areas of the body to help assure success when dealing with determined foe. For now, be aware that merely delivering pain may not be sufficient to control a situation.

Never Quit

On January 1, 2008, Meredith Emerson, a 24-year-old University of Georgia graduate, managed to fend off both a knife and a baton attack, holding her own until her assailant tricked her into surrendering. Gary Michael Hilton, a burly 61-year-old drifter, subsequently tied her up and carried her to a remote location where he raped and eventually killed her three days later.

Hilton reportedly told police interrogators that his petite victim nearly overpowered him when he first accosted her on an Appalachian hiking trail. According to published reports, Hilton stalked the 5-foot-4-inch tall, 120-pound woman on the trail but was unable to keep up so he laid in wait and intercepted her on her way back down. He pulled a knife and demanded her ATM card. Emerson, a trained martial artist, recognized the threat and immediately fought back.

"I lost control, and she fought. And as I read in the paper, she's a martial artist." Emerson, who held middle kyu ranks (blue belt and green belt) in two different martial arts, ripped the knife out of his hands. He countered with a baton that she was also able

> to pull from his grasp. As the struggle continued, they fell down a steep slope, leaving both weapons behind. "The bayonet is probably still up there," Hilton later told investigators.
>
> "I had to hand-fight her," Hilton said. "She wouldn't stop fighting and yelling at the same time so I needed to both control her and silence her." He kept punching her, blackening her eyes, fracturing her nose, and breaking his own hand in the process. He figured that he had worn her down as they moved farther off the trail, but suddenly she began fighting again. He finally got her to stop by telling her that all he wanted was her credit card and PIN number.
>
> Once she relaxed her guard, he restrained her hands with a zip tie, took her to a remote location, and tied her to a tree. Predators often take their victims to secondary crime scenes where they have the privacy to perform their depravations. Sadly this was no exception. He kept her captive in the wilderness for three terrifying days before telling her that he was ready to let her go.
>
> Then he beat her to death with a car-jack handle and cut off her head.
>
> Hilton made a plea deal with prosecutors, leading investigators to his victim's remains so that they would not seek the death penalty for his crimes. He was subsequently sentenced to life in prison with the possibility of parole after 30 years.

The goal of self-defense is not to win a fight, but rather to avoid combat in the first place. After all, the only battle you are guaranteed to walk away from unscathed is the one you never engage in. Taking a beat-down can seriously mess up your life. Nevertheless, sometimes despite your best intentions, you may find yourself in a situation where there really is no alternative but to fight. When it comes to such circumstances, particularly in an asocial violence scenario, you cannot stop until it's over.

Once engaged in battle, it is critical to remain mentally and physically prepared to fight or continue a brawl at a moment's notice. Always keep your opponent in sight until you can escape to safety. Even if your blow knocks an adversary to the ground, remain alert for a possible continuation of his attack. Most fistfights end when one combatant gives up rather than when he or she can no longer physically continue. Weapons bring a whole new dynamic into play. Even fatally wounded adversaries do not always succumb to their injuries right away; they can continue to be a critical danger for several seconds, if not minutes. That is a very long time in a fight.

Never give up until you are sure that you are safe. Sadly, too many victims do not heed this lesson, with tragic results.

Never believe anything an assailant tells you. His actions have already demonstrated beyond any doubt that he's a bad guy. Do not relax your guard and get caught by surprise; that is a good way to die. If the other guy thinks that he is losing, he might be more inclined to play possum or pull out a weapon in order to cheat to win. Worse yet, street attacks sometimes involve multiple assailants, many of whom may be seasoned fighters who know how to take a blow and shrug off the pain. Be mindful of additional assailants, potentially latecomers, and be prepared to continue your defense as long as necessary.

As the Chinese proverb states, "Dead tigers kill the most hunters." Remain vigilant during any pause in the fight. You may be facing multiple assailants, an adversary who pulls a weapon in the middle of a fight, or an opponent who just won't quit. Once you have removed yourself from the danger and are absolutely certain that you are no longer under threat, you can safely begin to relax your guard.

Account for Adrenaline

When I took a defensive handgun course several years ago, I was taught to train for handling the survival-stress reaction commonly associated with actual combat. To simulate the reaction, we had to do as many pushups as we could as fast as we could for one minute. Immediately after completing the pushups, we sprinted to the parking lot and raced around the building four times as fast as we could go, covering close to a mile in the process. We then sprinted back into the building and attempted to accurately fire down range under the watchful eye of our instructors.

While I could normally hit the bulls-eye of a static paper target much of the time at 25 feet during shooting competitions, and always put every shot in the black, the first time I attempted to do so after this stress test, I missed the paper completely. It was an eye-opening experience.

When adrenaline courses through your system during a fight, you can be stabbed, shot, or badly mangled and yet persevere, at least until the pain kicks in afterward. Your ability to think rationally is greatly reduced. The good news is that you tend to become stronger and more resilient than usual. The bad news, however, is that you will likely have degraded motor skills, experience tunnel vision, and perhaps even suffer temporary hearing or memory loss.

While precise movements are extraordinarily tough, even imprecise ones like grabbing a wrist or hooking a leg can be problematic even if you are highly trained. If you try to get too fancy, you will hurt your chances for success in a fight. However, gross motor movements, especially those that target vital areas of the adversary's body, can work pretty well.

The more comprehensive and realistic your training is, the better you will perform in actual combat because conditioned responses can help you counteract, or at least work through, the effects of adrenaline. Conversely, the more stressed you are through exertion, fear, or desperation, the harder it is perform. Mostly. A friend of ours, who hijacks planes (from terrorists) for a living, puts it this way:

"The body's reaction under critical incident stress has almost nothing to do with how you think rationally. Instead, it has almost everything has to do with ingrained responses, be they trained ones or instinctive ones. The amygdala will choose. It has the chemical authority to override your conscious thoughts and decisions.

"It also has the chemical authority to enforce its decision despite your conscious will. This is why divers are found drowned yet with full oxygen tanks—something happened to them and the amygdala reacted to that critical incident stress with its preferred strategy—clearing obstructions from the breathing passage. As a

general rule, getting stuff out of your mouth is an excellent strategy for a land-based species in land-based confrontations. But spitting out your breathing tube is a terrible strategy under water. The fact is none of those drowning victims really thought they could breathe water. Something happened and their bodies reacted.

"Like a diver in duress, when you face a threat on the street you won't be doing much thinking. Unless you have a very high adrenal threshold and/or a LOT of training. Deliberate thought is slow, taking several seconds to accomplish. That's an eternity in a critical incident. Might as well go get a massage while you're at it...

"Deeply ingrained reactions are far more likely than conscious decisions. And don't even get me started on how much training you have to do to override and replace your body's instinctive responses with new ones. Regardless, you won't be selecting an option from a menu of choices calmly and rationally like you do in the training hall. Your body is going to pick its own response in a maelstrom of shit and adrenaline.

"Training then, to me, is all about trying to give the amygdala better choices. Because you won't consciously be deciding on much on 'that day.' Or maybe it's about getting your body so used to adrenal stress that you can actually think, somewhat, during pauses in the action. Or more likely a combination of the two. End of the day, training isn't about what most people think it is."

—M. Guthrie, Federal Air Marshal

As Bruce Siddle described in his book, *Sharpening the Warrior's Edge*, in a violent encounter your heart rate can jump from 60 or 70 beats per minute (BPM) to well over 200 BMP in less than half a second. Elevated heart rate is an easily measurable symptom of the effects of adrenaline, one that can be used to index what happens to you when adrenalized:

- For people whose resting heart rate is around 60 to 70 BPM, at around 115 BPM many begin to lose fine motor skills such as

finger dexterity making it difficult to successfully dial a phone, open a lock, or aim a weapon.
- Around 145 BPM most people begin to lose their complex motor skills such as hand-eye coordination, precise tracking movements, or exact timing, making complicated techniques very challenging if not impossible.
- Around 175 BPM most people begin to lose depth perception, experience tunnel vision, and sometimes even suffer temporary memory loss.
- Around 185–220 BPM many people experience hypervigilance, loss of rational thought, and inability to consciously move or react. Without prior training, the vast majority of people cannot function at this stress level.

Breath control techniques can help you minimize or recover from the effects of adrenaline, particularly if you have enough time to see an attack coming. Begin by breathing in through the nose and out through the mouth following a 4-count process for each step—inhalation, hold, exhalation, hold. In other words, each cycle of combat breathing includes:

- Inhale for a 4-count.
- Hold for a 4-count.
- Exhale for a 4-count.
- Hold for a 4-count with empty lungs.

When men are confronted with extreme emotional or violent situations, their adrenaline kicks off like a rocket, surging quickly and then dissipating rapidly afterward as well. In a home invasion situation, for example, when the male homeowner shoots the suspect, the killing is likely to take place near the front door. When police officers arrive, they will typically find that the suspect has been shot perhaps two or three times, just enough to make sure he is no longer a threat.

Women, on the other hand, get a much slower, longer-lasting adrenaline surge. It takes longer to get going and dissipates a lot more slowly than you find in men. In that same home invasion scenario, police often find the dead robber in a back bedroom where he had chased and cornered the female homeowner. But here's the kicker.

Rather than shooting him a couple of times, she's emptied the gun into him, perhaps even reloading and doing it again.

Interesting difference, huh? An implication is that women have more time to think, but must often defend themselves before becoming adrenalized, whereas men get the advantages and disadvantages of adrenaline without the clear-headed ability to plan.

It's NOT a Continuum

The rest of the book lays out several levels of force in a logical order, covering (1) presence, (2) voice, (3) touch, (4) empty-hand/ physical restraint, (5) less-lethal force, and (6) lethal force. This by no means implies that these levels are stages on a ladder where you must move from one to another. Select the level you need to safely prevail/ escape. If your choice is not working, you may have to change levels quickly.

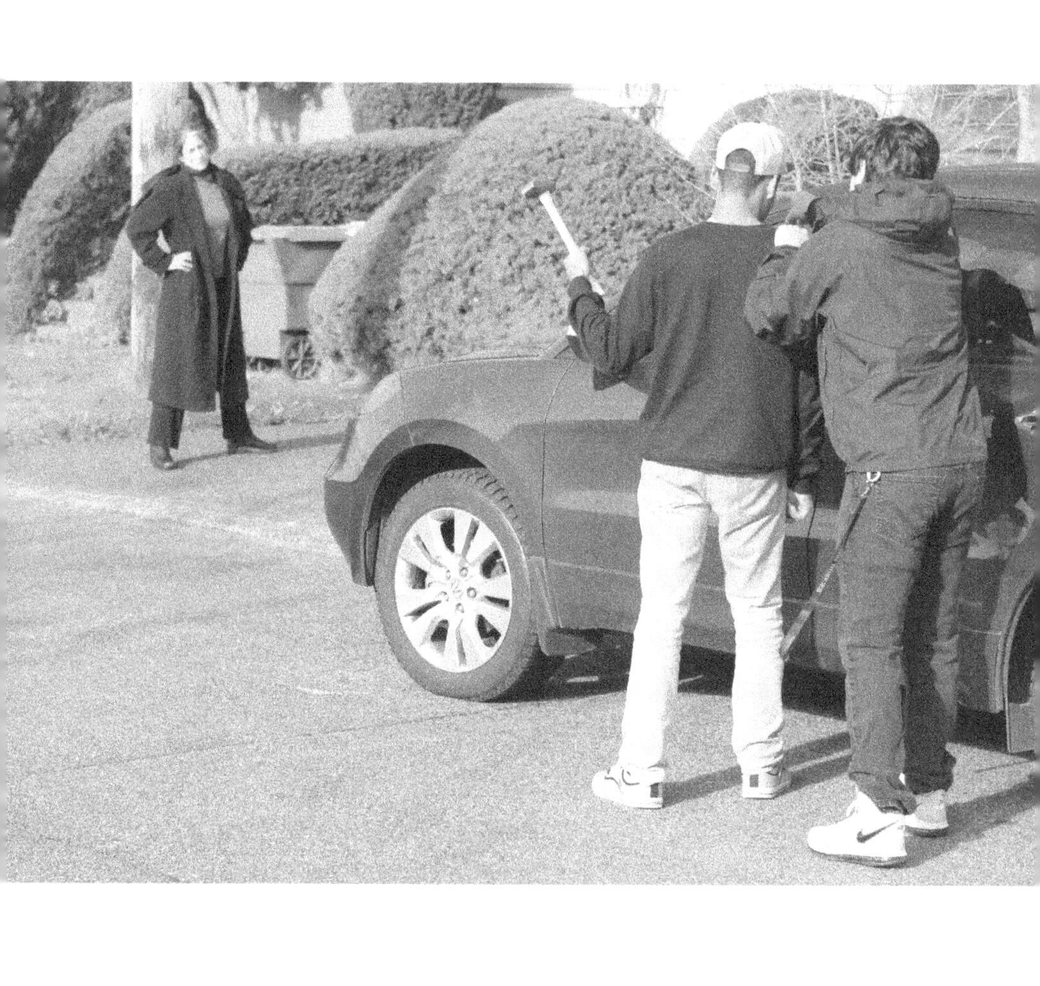

LEVEL 1—PRESENCE

Skillfully doing nothing.

Level 1 and Level 2 (presence and verbal) and to a lesser extent Level 3 (touch) are intended to make the threat quit being threatening without anyone getting hurt. While higher levels of force are aimed at an adversary's body, the lower levels work through the threat's mind.

In social violence, presence and verbal skills primarily aim at preventing or diverting the attention of someone who wants to monkey dance. Normally, that is easy—just don't play. Walk away. Disregard the challenge. Don't get caught in your own little monkey brain.

In asocial or predatory violence, particularly in a predatory ambush, the purpose of presence and verbal skills is to keep you off the victim list. As such they must become habits. You may never even know if they worked. If a predator scans you—which will happen several times a day in the crowded part of a big city—and decides to pass, chances are good that you will not even notice. Success, in this subject, is often invisible. If your habits of presence—how you walk, how you scan, what you do with positioning and your hands—are good, the bad guy quietly moves on, never even coming to your attention.

If you are under assault, it is too late to apply Levels 1 and 2 as primary techniques. Go ahead and scream, "Let me go!" while fighting back to help create witnesses sympathetic to your cause, but don't be stupid enough to scream *instead* of fighting back. If you are in danger and taking damage, you must be working from much higher up on the force scale than verbals.

These two lowest levels (and the third level, touch) often come into play when intervening as a third party. That does not always mean breaking up a fight. The simple presence of potential witnesses can prevent much crime. More so if the witness looks like he or she is paying attention or dialing a cell phone.

Generally, your goal with presence and verbal skills will be:

- To raise the stakes. The presence of witnesses or involved citizens may make committing a crime too risky.
- To give the threat a face-saving way to leave. If the threat has ego invested in his bad act, he may be afraid that walking away will make him look afraid. However, walking away from a group or a uniform or whispered advice that the police are on the way is often acceptable.
- To instill doubt. This can be a very effective strategy in that if the threat does not know who you are or what you are likely to do, he cannot be sure what the outcome of his actions will be.
- To give the threat a better choice. Sometimes you can get past the emotion and show the threat that his actions will not achieve his goals.

The Lowest Level of Force

On the second of September 2008, I did something stupid. I hadn't quite been in Iraq for two months and was still very much a rookie. Lawrence wants me to write down the story because there might be some lessons about presence in there. I'm reluctant for a couple of reasons and the reasons are important:

1. Lots of things that sound cool happened because there wasn't a good choice. That doesn't mean it was a good strategy. Rats don't swim very well—they only abandon a ship because sinking with it is worse.
2. Because something worked once, especially when the stakes were high, does not make it a good idea. The fear with anything that makes amateurs' eyes get all shiny is that they might try to do it. I wouldn't do this again if I had any choice.
3. I especially hate telling this story because though amateurs might think it's cool, every professional will read this and automatically (and correctly) label me as an idiot. I don't like being labeled an idiot, especially by people I respect.

But, Lawrence twisted my arm, so here goes...

The Records area at Rusafa Prison Complex in Baghdad is enclosed by a chain-link fence and was almost always crowded. It's a stressful place, with inmates being processed in and out, Iraqi military, police, corrections, advocates, politicos, and sometimes families of the convicts are present and a small handful of American advisors. It was especially crowded that day. Suddenly I heard a loud argument. I couldn't understand what was being shouted, but it was getting really loud.

I quickly discovered that two armed Iraqi gentleman were about to go at it. And no one was doing anything. Not the Iraqi officers and not the other Americans, all of whom were backing off.

This is what I do, right? I'm a freaking jail guard and my primary job is to prevent fights.

There were a ton of other considerations as well. First and foremost, I only spoke about fifty words of Arabic and almost all of them were either formal greetings or commands, neither of which was appropriate for this situation. You do not yell commands at people you want to calm down. Second, I had no formal authority—I was an advisor and mentor. Third, I had no idea what the argument was about. And, I didn't know who the guys involved were. They could have been department ministers, tribal leaders, or just about anything else. That means that I didn't know what would happen if things got messy. Would it stay personal or get really big?

Other than the language barrier (and the weapons), this is what corrections officers deal with all the time. This is the regular job. Usually I can call for backup first and know it is on the way, but not today...

There were two other factors that I thought were very important. The biggest was that if things got really out of hand, we were all screwed. I could handle two people. But if one pulled a gun and the other responded and a few friends got involved and the armed security guys got nervous, there would be a bloodbath inside a chain-link enclosed area. The second was probably less logical, but important to me. The Iraqi officers we advised were under a lot of pressure from criminals, militias, and secretly loyal members of the old regime. They were not paid very much and were constantly being threatened or tempted by bribes. One of our primary missions was to teach them to stand on principle, do the right thing. It was dangerous and took a lot of guts for them to avoid corruption, more so because they were coming off thirty years of totalitarian rule where anyone who showed a spine was summarily executed.

It was probably illogical, but I thought it would be tragic if they saw all of the American advisors back down from a dangerous situation.

So I stepped in. Got between the two fighters, squaring off with the biggest, invading his space, smiling slightly but with eyes calm, talking softly and low-pitched.

It takes a lot to invade an Arab's space; culturally it's much closer than Westerners'. He started moving when I put my chest against his arms and pressed with a step. All of this happened while I had a hand poised in the place he couldn't see behind his arm, ready to control the leverage point on the back of the elbow and spin him if I had to. DON'T EVEN CONSIDER close range de-escalation unless you have absolute confidence in your infighting skills and can take an invisible position of advantage.

I took a step forward, he took one back. In a few seconds, he was outside of the enclosure.

Then the other guy got in a beef with someone else.

I'd chosen the biggest, but he evidently wasn't the one starting the problem. So I used the same method to get the other guy out, diffusing the situation.

My boss's boss and I had a private talk within the hour:

> "You do not, for any reason, go into a group of armed Iraqis."
> "Yes sir."
> "You do not, except in self-defense, lay hands on an Iraqi."
> "But I didn't...yes sir."
> "You do not, ever risk your own life just to make a point."

Right there, he had me. That's the lesson I want you to take from this incident and the whole book. I don't care how cool it sounds.

> Risking your life for anything other than saving a life is ego, it's bullshit, and it is childish.

Presence is the lowest level of force—not force at all if you think in terms of mechanical power—and it comes just from being there. If presence works, it is a perfect solution: no paperwork, no one gets hurt, and you don't even have to talk to the guy.

Even if presence does not work by itself, it makes every other level of the force continuum a little easier. An order given by someone who looks like an officer or a mother works better than a pimply teenager trying to take control. You will feel the difference between a wrist-lock done with authority and one attempted with a lack of confidence. Using a stick like you know what you are doing is more likely to get a threat to back down than if you look like you are not sure how to hold it.

Even at the lethal force level, there is a qualitative difference between a professional about to use a gun as a tool and a scared civilian trying to hide behind a weapon.

There is no downside to developing presence. That said, because it is so subjective, it can be damnably hard to develop. What follows are a few small hints on a very big subject...

The Intangibles

We are going to get all metaphysical for a second and talk about stuff that everyone knows but that we often pretend is too mystical to acknowledge.

A big part of your presence is who you are. An asshole carries himself like an asshole and almost everyone can sense who and what he is. Curious people look like curious people. Someone with a good heart makes other people relax, even if the people relaxing can never really explain why.

Some can fake it—conmen are famous for it, but even conmen don't run games on certain people. It just does not work.

In what follows, take that into account. A smaller person intimidates differently than a bigger one does, even if they are equally competent. Men cannot pull off the "mom vibe" that can sometimes be even more effective than physical intimidation. Not all tactics work for all people. Bad things do not happen around some people because they have the kind of aura that makes people want to be good around them. Take Rory's wife Kami, for example. Folks seem to need her to approve of them and some big, rough, tough bad men call her "ma'am" and will be happy to do whatever she says. It's been that way for over twenty years.

Conversely, people tend to be good in Rory's presence because they sense that he will come down on them hard if they don't. Lawrence is adept at keeping drunken frat boys from doing incredibly stupid things, oftentimes without needing to say a word.

That is the very definition of presence in a force continuum—people often quit being bad when they see other people.

There is one more intangible concept that is tied up with presence, the martial arts concept of *zanshin*. Humans can sense the intensity of another human being. That intensity derives from both awareness and experience. The more you have been through, the greater your intensity, your presence. The more alert you are, the more you sense and perceive, the greater your presence.

But intensity is almost never the same as tension. Kids trying to look intense give a bug-eyed stare. Truly intense people tend to be calm, relaxed, and watchful, sometimes elaborately relaxed when everyone else is on the edge of panic.

Experience will come with time, but you can always practice being more aware.

The Power of Authority

There is a certain weight that we all have as humans. When someone is being bad and other people are watching, there is a glitch as the threat wonders how he looks. Humans are social primates and a lot of evolution went into developing concern about how other people perceive us.

It is not super strong. It is strongest in asocial violence where a witness is an immediate threat to the criminal's future. In social violence, witnesses may be the point. After all, you can't get a reputation without witnesses.

Just being there, however, gives a chance that the situation will defuse.

There are other factors that can add to this base. How these factors affect the outcome depend on interplay between the threat, the behavior, and what additional signals you bring to the table.

A uniformed officer, for instance, theoretically brings the whole authority of society along with him. Realistically, what an officer adds to the equation is someone who will not look the other way and pretend that nothing is happening. This makes the threat decide if his actions are worth the consequences—and understand this: Most bad guys resort to violence expecting to have no bad consequences, and they are usually right. Unless someone steps in (and is willing to risk all that comes on the line in a violent encounter), most low-level violence is rewarded, not punished. Civilians can, and often do, look the other way. A law enforcement officer, security guard, bouncer, or similar authority figure typically cannot (or is not supposed to, anyway).

Different societies treat authority very differently though. For example, in most of South and Central America, if you make direct eye contact with an officer, it's grounds for an immediate and potentially severe beating.

It is not just the uniform. Other people bring authority to the situation too, though not in the same way. In some areas, a little old lady is nearly the ultimate authority figure. This is because most of the bad elements in certain areas have been raised by their grandmothers. She is the one person who has earned their absolute respect. And love. A grandmother won't have the same automatic response from a kid who was raised where the grandparents were people you visited occasionally, got stuff from, and who let you do whatever you wanted.

Certain professions and certain situations have more weight of personality. Take members of the clergy, for example. Or medical personnel. In some countries there is no such thing as medical malpractice. Doctors can do pretty much whatever they want.

This kind of presence has its reverse side as well.

> Dark shades, a black tank-top, and tattered blue jeans, he gets on the train at one of the downtown stops next to the Parole and Probation Office. His name is tattooed on his neck, a teardrop tattooed under his eye, his gang affiliation on his shoulder. He has obviously been working out in prison until quite recently. Muscles ripple.
>
> The other passengers lower their voices and don't make eye contact, fearing to draw his attention.

Presence affects behavior without saying a word. It is not exclusively a tool for good guys or a way to prevent violence. People commit crimes without saying a word, through presence alone. If you turn away from the ATM with a handful of bills and see someone pointing a gun at you, does he need to say anything?

Fitness

We are going to work this from inside to outside. At the very core of who you are, one of the things that people see right away and one of the things that affects everything else about you is your level of fitness.

> I was still on probation about 4 months into the job, working dayshift in the East Side Jail. The sergeant came into my dorm to do rounds and stopped by the desk briefly. He then proceeded over toward the dayroom area and climbed on top of a bookshelf. He then somehow scaled up the wall and over the second-tier railing onto the second floor. I thought, "What the hell is this guy doing?" I continued to sit at my desk while he walked the second tier. When he came down he said, "See ya later," and left.
>
> From then on I knew he was a pretty unique guy…

Fitness is not the only thing, however. People mess with big guys and body-builders too. When Rory was working Casino security at 5'9" and maybe 150 pounds, no one swung on him. Thai, one of his partners, a big, fit college football player seemed to get swung on every week.

The math was simple—where's the glory in beating up a little kid? Conversely, someone tees off on the little guy and loses; he just got his ass kicked by a kid. That's not good. Swing on the big guy, however, and it's big points if you win. Even if you lose, you get a reputation for heart. In this example, a contributing factor may have been that too many folks knew that Thai was very professional. He would do everything in his power not to injure anyone.

That's target acquisition for social violence, though.

Fitness and size really pay off when you show up as a witness or bystander to a predatory crime. The threat did not choose you for the mathematics of reputation. He was doing something else. You are now screwing up his plan and the general perception is that big people can screw up plans better than small people.

The best part about fitness is what it does to the rest of you. The more you use your body, the more you play with it and test it, the more at home you feel inside it. The more comfortable you are and the more comfortable you look. That is a step toward remaining calm in the face of adversity. Composure is one of the signs that you know what you are doing.

Even if you have no idea what you are doing, looking calm makes people think twice about pushing you. That's a payoff, one which you can easily throw away by hopping from foot to foot and looking nervous.

Fitness also does not hurt if things go physical, of course. Size and strength aren't everything, but they do help. A lot.

Fitness does not always mean size and strength. People inexperienced at violence look at size first, muscle definition second. Experienced people look at movement. When the sergeant scaled the wall to the second level, he not only showed the inmates some serious physicality, but also tremendous functional strength and a habit of moving and thinking unconventionally. Climbing is a great test and demonstration of functional strength. The combined message was one of physical effectiveness and unpredictability, a combination most experienced street-fighters seek to avoid.

It's easy enough to say "work out."

So we will: Go work out.

But you probably want specifics:

- Do something you enjoy. If you have to make yourself go, it's easy to quit.
- Do something with unpredictable requirements. Grappling or rock climbing or swimming in rivers or oceans puts unpredictable loads on you that make you adapt. That is good training so long as you do it safely.
- Total body movement should be a huge element of training. Climbing and grappling uses total body movement, but basketball and soccer are also excellent for this kind of training. Move your whole body. Isolation work is great for building a chiseled physique, but in real life, especially in a violent encounter, you will need to use your whole body. Practice now.
- Aerobic exercise is the king for health maintenance, but fighting for your life is profoundly anaerobic. Make sure you work your anaerobic system hard.
- Practice something that does not let you decide to quit. Grappling matches do not let you quit when you want to, unless you like losing. The same concept applies to free solo rock climbing—you can't just quit forty feet up. The basketball or soccer game goes until the time runs out. Even milking a cow or baling hay, you don't get to quit until the job is done. That is an important element to training, especially going to complete muscle failure and having to find a way to continue.
- Try to limit injuries. Injuries are counterproductive and you will regret them in a decade or so. Perhaps earlier. That is why even though rugby can be far better for combat conditioning than almost any other sport, we don't recommend it officially.
- Do something that requires strength, speed, endurance, and flexibility. Do not do exercises for each area, but rather do something, like (again) climbing or grappling or soccer or football where you need all these attributes to excel. It is the best incentive to develop a balanced physicality.

Posture and Stance

Posture is how you stand. You probably got "Stand up straight!" from your parents and little else. Maybe you got the "Chin up, shoulders back, belly in." Maybe you got a martial arts instructor's "Eyes forward, shoulders square, tuck your tail bone under, etc."

It does not matter. Most of what matters with posture comes from fitness or grace, an ability to be comfortable in your body. A coordinated, athletic person who walks slightly hunched over gives the impression of being coiled. An un-athletic person with similar body language looks timid. An athlete standing up straight looks alert and "soldierly" while a schmoe looks stiff and awkward. You get the idea.

That is basic posture. Stance is another concept altogether. Stance is how you set and prepare your body. Posture tells something about your underlying health. Stance says something about your personality.

"I thought that was going to go bad," Mike said.

"Why?"

"Because you do that thing that you always do just before someone hits the floor." Mike turned to face me and sort of crossed his arms, left hand across his ribs, right elbow resting on his left hand, right fingers scratching his eyebrow. "Like that. You do that when you're talking someone down but when your right wrist cocks back, you're about to launch."

I don't know whether I was disturbed or happy that the second in command of my tactical team watched me that closely. "Well, it didn't go bad."

"Yeah, he sensed it. He backed right down."

That stance is sometimes called the Modified Columbo after Peter Falk's character in the television show. It has good protection, yet you can launch any number of pre-emptive or reactionary attacks. And it doesn't look threatening. At least, not until your friends and the bad guys start telling stories about you.

We suggest that you have two preparatory stances.

One is for when you think things might go bad. Your "spidey sense" tingles or you get a bad feeling or you are talking to someone who appears agitated but not overtly threatening or aggressive. This stance should have good static defense—if you get sucker punched, you cannot count on having time to react. You should have mobility to close, angle forward, or angle back. You should be able to attack from the stance. Possibly most important, the stance should not look threatening to the uninitiated in any way.

The next stance is for when things are going bad. It should have all the same physical advantages as the preparatory stance but can be more overt. You can fight from the Modified Columbo directly, but sometimes it is valuable to take it a step up.

Violence is a form of communication. Shifting to a ready combat stance is sending the signal one last time that you are ready and giving the threat time to change his mind. Continuing the previous example, keep your hands open and palms toward the threat. Part of that is pragmatic—it facilitates grips and infighting. Part is that it will remind witnesses that you were not the aggressor, a benefit that is lost with closed fists.

Lastly, because it still looks placating rather than challenging, BUT shows that the risk has escalated, it BOTH gives the threat additional incentive to change his mind AND a face-saving way out. This is key. With closed fists, the other guy feels like he is backing down. His ego might not let him do that. Keeping the hands open, on the other hand, he can convince himself that he showed mercy. Pretty slick, huh?

The first step for training stances is to look at yourself in a mirror. How would you attack someone in that stance? What are your vulnerabilities? Also pay attention to your expression. You may not project the emotion and intent that you think you do. Try to look angry, thoughtful, or serious and see if the look in the mirror matches the one in your head.

Then practice moving from the stance. The stances most commonly used by an art say a lot about the style, predilections for distance, angle, and applications when it

We're not talking about stances as they are commonly taught in the martial arts. Traditional stances are incredibly valuable, but generally misunderstood and mistaught. The classic stances—front, back, horse, etc., are positions of remarkable power. Use your own falling body weight to damage or unbalance an adversary and you will almost certainly catch yourself in one of the classic stances. Your legs will be ballistically loaded to explode out of it and deliver damage on the opposite vector. Very neat. Not for standing in and trying to look cool. These postures are dynamic—you enter them while performing some kind of martial application.

comes to fighting. For infighters, the most critical movement is closing at an angle. Strikers need to control distance, so the most critical skill will be angling backward, going right or left rear. Not straight back—you probably can't move backward as fast as the bad guy can move forward. If you are an aggressive, close-range fighter, a straight close may work for you. It depends on both the style you practice as well as your demeanor.

We'll talk about proxemics, how you stand in relationship to another person, later, but watch your range. That means different things to different people. Infighters who have much experience reading pre-assault cues tend to work much closer than most folks should. Out of reach is usually a good idea.

Lastly, practice counterattacking from the stance. This is usually best in armor—counterassault training should be done at speed and you should take care not to pull punches. Technically, counterassault should be conditioned, not trained. From your preparatory stance, such as the Modified Columbo, your partner tries to sucker punch you. You counterattack at the first hint of movement.

At first you will get clocked. A lot. That's good because one of the things you will learn is that getting hit, especially if you are moving, is not a big, scary, dangerous thing. We occasionally run into black belts in striking arts who have never been hit in the face. That's troubling.

Appearance and Demeanor

Appearance is what you look like. Demeanor is what you try to look like your expression. There are some things you cannot change. For example, taller people are automatically given more respect than short people. That's the way it is, whether you like it or not. Women are generally treated with more deference than men; men with more respect (even when women are shown deference, such as opening doors, it is sometimes patronizing). Athletic people are taken more seriously than the obese. A statement from an older person is automatically given more weight than a statement from a child, unless the oldster is too old.

Pretty people are treated better than ugly people. This all may suck. And sound unfair. It is unfair like much of the natural world. But we all have to deal with it. There's nothing you can do about some aspects of your appearance. Height and coloration and well...pretty much height and coloration. Almost anything else you can affect to some degree.

> The newest rookie was tiny—short, slender with thick glasses. I looked over at Ralph, "The new kid is going to have a rough time."
>
> "Yeah, he'll either have it or he won't. If he can hack it, get a rep, he'll be good."
>
> The kid stuck it out. His first year was hell, constantly challenged, but Ralph was right. The kid had some steel.

The most important thing you can do is to be healthy. Physical appearance, specifically beauty, is based almost entirely on a few clues as to general health. Height/weight proportionate. Smooth skin. Clear eyes. Hair sheen. Scent. All of these things can be affected to varying degrees. Some people struggle with weight—if the advantages are worth the lifestyle change, go for it. Otherwise, don't.

Skin, hair, eyes, and scent are profoundly affected by two things: nutrition and hygiene. Want clear skin? Eat right; lots of fresh (preferably raw) fruits and vegetables, protein, and stay entirely away from sugar. Then wash with soap and water. Frequently. Works for scent as well. Add regular exercise and it works for weight. Stay away from drugs and alcohol, and get adequate sleep and fresh air, and the eyes stay bright and clear.

The things you cannot change, height and coloration, can work for you or against you. We have a saying: "The difference between a hazard and a tool is who uses it first."

Height, except at the extremes, can be psychologically enhanced or minimized. A short person with good posture (in your parent's "stand up straight" definition) looks taller than a big person with bad posture. Choices of clothing can change the perceived height and weight of people.

Consciously or unconsciously, shy tall people tend to have bad posture, a way of looking smaller and drawing less attention. Short people often stand on curbs to look taller and many tall people like to sit when they talk to set people at ease.

Your style—the verbal and presence skills that you develop—will be affected by conditions you cannot change. If you were born tall and imposing, it's useful to practice relaxing others by looking inoffensive. But it is important to practice intimidation, too. Mother Nature gave you a leg up. Use it.

> An old boss, one of the best I'd ever seen at talking a drunk out of fighting, was amazing at his job. I asked him how he learned to do it.
>
> "Well, son, it was all about girls. About the time I was your age, I really wanted to go out with a lot of girls. So I took a long look at myself in the mirror and I said to myself, 'Boy, looks like you're gonna have to be a talker.'"

Small people can develop some skills that take advantage of their size. Take walking quietly, for instance. A relatively small guy, who suddenly appears out of nowhere, even if he is friendly, can make bad people rethink their plans.

Hair and eye coloration can be changed. Generally, hair coloring should be subtle. Specific changes in appearance that draw attention or seem intended to draw attention send very specific messages. Sadly, it's rarely the message that the person intended. Facial tats or eye-blowing hair color intended to shout, "I'm an individual!" are usually (almost universally) interpreted as, "What underlying insecurity caused such a pathetic plea for attention?"

Eye color can be changed via cosmetic contact lenses if you really want to go that route. Skin coloring is harder to change. Any skin color can be an advantage or a disadvantage depending on the audience and how you play it.

Demeanor, expression, is our primary means of communicating emotion and intention to others. Not words, demeanor. If someone is crying and says, "I'm fine. Everything is fine," we do not trust the words. Expression is king. That means, for the most part, most people are pretty good at reading expressions. It also means that most people are terrible at lying with their expressions and body language.

Lying? Is that too loaded a word? In a conflict situation, you may feel fear or nervousness. Those are not, generally, the message you want to send. The feelings you choose to project may not be what you actually feel. So you can pretty up the language any way you want, but we are talking about lying with body language.

In some situations that is a very valuable skill. The reason that most people are poor at it has nothing to do with evolution or some mystical need to communicate emotional truths. It is really as simple as the fact that most people don't look at themselves when they are talking. Use a video camera or simply practice in front of a mirror. Actors become good at it. So can you.

Choose an expression and try it on yourself in a mirror. It may not look like it feels. For example, one of Rory's students used to practice a tough guy stare. Because he felt tension around his eyes and his mouth, he thought it was a hard glare. From outside, the twisted up eyes and white lips looked like a child trying not to cry. Clearly not what he wanted to project.

Practice your expressions and your body language. They will be stilted at first—that's the difference between a good actor and a bad one, practice or take an acting class. If possible, video some of your regular interactions and "read" yourself. Watch the legalities of this though. It's possible that when you think you are projecting confidence, you are projecting something very different.

Attire

How you dress tells a lot about you. Look at shoes. People usually buy the best shoes they can afford, so their footwear not only suggests a lot about their socioeconomic level, but also what is important to them. Is it a fashion statement or something that is comfortable to walk in? Steel toed and non-slip? Flip-flops?

> One couple came in with three kids, one a babe in arms and two young boys. Black hair, dark eyes, olive skin—this station serves a

relatively heavily Hispanic neighborhood but the vibe wasn't quite right.

I glanced at the woman's shoes and there it was—an Arabic family. I eavesdropped shamelessly. I wasn't sure about the accent at first, a couple of hundred words in Iraqi Arabic hardly qualifies me as a linguist, but I caught part of a slang term, "shaku maku" and I was pretty sure.

The man was dressed in beige 5.11 pants, the unofficial uniform of the contractors working over there. I was wearing a pair myself.

Clothing has a lot of impact as a message. It can tell people about your ethnic origin, (*hijab*, *keffiyeh*, *tartan*) give hints to your religion (*yarmulke*, crucifix, Thor's hammer), and your economic status (Wrangler, Levis, Jordache). It can indicate membership in a group (red or blue scarves, Masonic rings). It can tell your profession (5.11 pants and an untucked shirt, surgical scrubs).

It can even indicate something about your values—is comfort more important than appearance? Is it more important to blend in or stand out?

Does this have a lot to do with presence? It can, but aside from a few jobs (most of which provide a uniform anyway) using your presence to prevent bad things is not realistically going to be the primary reason to choose clothing.

It doesn't hurt, though, to be aware of what you are projecting, especially if what you are actually projecting is very different from what you wish. Each generation has a rebellious group who want to be different and individuals who all seem to wind up looking the same. Okay if that is your intent. Sad if it is not.

Here is one piece of very good, but possibly expensive advice for you. It is especially useful if you rarely think about personal style or have trouble getting attention from the opposite sex.

Save up about a month's worth of wages. Then get one or two good friends of the opposite sex to take you shopping. They are to get your hair cut or styled and pick out clothes for you. Your job is to keep your mouth shut and trust their judgment. Having an idealized version of what you could look like sets a goal and opens up new opportunity.

Behavior

So far, presence has all been about how you appear. It is time to talk about what you are going to do. Remember that the goal at this level is not to hurt anyone. You don't even go hands on. Going hands on when you do not need to is "excessive force." This information will interact powerfully with all that has gone before and the next section on positioning. Nothing stands alone; nothing works in a vacuum.

> The young, aggressive inmate had somehow managed to get assigned to a dorm with primarily vulnerable inmates—some very old, many mentally ill. It was like a shark in a goldfish bowl. The officer on duty had received a lot of complaints, but hadn't caught him violating a rule. It might be days before we could arrange to move him to a housing unit with a tougher victim pool.
>
> I went up the little shark's cell and keyed my way in. I didn't say a word.
>
> "Hey, you can't just come in here."
>
> He was wrong about that. I didn't say a word. I started looking through his property, through his books.
>
> "If this is about that candy bar, the old man gave me that. I didn't take it. No matter what he told you." Still no answer. I picked a book from his collection and started reading it. He got more and more nervous. Most people don't deal with silence very well.
>
> I put the book down after a few minutes and left. Never said a word.
>
> Had we been dogs, I would have pissed in every corner of his cell. The effect, and the message, was the same. This was my territory, not his. He was not the big dog. By acting so far outside his experience of how people should act, he became uncertain. He could no longer calculate the costs and benefits of his own actions.
>
> The dorm, as a result, was much quieter and much safer.

Behavior, appearance, and speech interact. Sometimes silence is communication as well. When it is, your behavior has to rise to the level of performance art. Communication is about getting a message or impression from your head into the other person's. With or without words, that takes practice.

Lots of things come out naturally in your behavior—your physicality, your comfort with yourself, how you feel about people. That's just in the way you move. How you stand shows whether you are prepared or unprepared, if you are on top of things or lax. It also shows exactly what you think of the person you are addressing:

- Ignoring someone indicates that they are unworthy of your attention.
- Eye contact and a stance readied to move forward indicate that you see a challenge.
- Likewise with hands up or forward, you perceive a threat.
- Focus on the face, but not particularly the eyes, shows interest.
- Combined with an open stance, shows trust (possibly misplaced).

The list goes on. The hard part with teaching yourself to influence others through behavior is that everything is a matter of degree. Restless movement can be read as eagerness. Or as nervous fear. Relaxed body language can seem a sign of cool competence or of ignorance or laziness. This aspect has come up before in this section but it bears repeating here—inside your own head is not the place to figure out how you look to others.

Watch videos of yourself. Listen to your recorded voice. The best advances either of us made were in instructor development courses where experienced teachers dissected our teaching and presentation styles. They were not only able to say what we failed to get across or how our behaviors distracted students, but specifically what action(s) caused what reaction.

You will find, like many skills—breathing, walking, talking, or writing, to name a few—that when everyone does it to some degree, most think that they do it well. That's simply not true. In each of these skills, you will find professionals who do have a system and practice the skill at a much higher, much more conscious level. The professionals for this skill are high-end teachers and actors.

There are additional things you can do to work projecting what you want to, other than taking acting classes:

- Watch animals, particularly pack animals like dogs. Animals don't have the luxury of speech and do most of their communication through behavior. Watch, learn, and interpret. Then pick up some books on canine behavior for explanations. You will find much of it applies to people.
- While you are at it, pick up some books on how monkeys behave in the wild. You'll be amazed how many of the behaviors you spot in your friends and classmates or co-workers.
- Watch some old black-and-white movies. Look for where the actor is trying to send a specific message or make an impression. Break down how he does this. In the silent-film era, there were specific gestures and stances that made an emotional language of sorts. These still have power today.
- Watch yourself and get honest feedback. If someone says you look nervous or tired or upset, ask what specifically makes you look that way. It's not just demeanor, it will also be the way you stand and move and what you do.

Positioning and Proxemics

Positioning and proxemics (how you stand in relationship to another human) are how you control space. The U.S. Marine Corps (USMC) advocates maneuver warfare, being in the perfect place at the perfect time so that the enemy is aware they have no chance.

The training scenario was to rescue an officer down who was covered by a barricaded bad guy. Danny played the bad guy and he had a metal desk for cover at the end of a long hallway, a classic "funnel of death." Even against a snatch team of four SWAT officers, Danny had the advantage.

It took us two days of brainstorming before we figured out how to storm that hallway with a good chance of success.

No, I'm not going to tell you how.

Three of the keys of positioning are the ability to (1) control a space, (2) observe a space, and (3) access escape routes. It is hard to physically control a large space without weapons, but this section is about presence anyway, not weapons. The advantage of thinking this way, choosing your position with respect to power, is that the most experienced violent people will recognize what you did. They will not know if you are armed or not; it is generally a foolish thing to confirm or deny, but they will take note. And it will affect their behavior.

The position of physical dominance should also be a place where people cannot easily reach you. It is subconscious, perhaps, but the big desk in the company president's office or the podium in front of the speaker are barriers and dead zones. They create shields between the person in the power position and everyone else. They are also placed facing, for the most part, the entrance(s) and the majority of the people. The guy at the podium is almost always in a power position.

The same point in a room also tends to give the best observational advantage. You should choose a place that allows you to see as much of the room as possible, especially as many entrances as possible. Ideally, it should be difficult for people to get behind you.

The third element is available escape routes. Being ready to fight is one skill. Being ready to run is another. Being ready to do either is just plain practical.

Positioning tactically augments your presence because it looks like you know what you are doing. Much of presence is an air of competence. The more competence you develop, the more presence you will show. Nor is this just an abstract game. The ideas that we talk about here can have huge payoffs when and if a situation goes bad.

Officers may need to dominate a room with their weapons. They must be in the right position to accomplish this. Being in that position, for that reason, sends a signal that makes bad things less likely to happen. A citizen positioned with an eye toward escape routes may be doing it as part of his program to look tough, but that escape route will become damnably handy if some disgruntled former employee walks in blasting away.

Presence on one level is a show, but you do not do these things for show. That is a side benefit.

Where you stand can also augment different aspects of your chosen style of presence. If you are going for quiet and unobtrusive, you may look for places where you are hidden from the power points in a room. If you want to be seen as more commanding, you can try for places that make you look taller.

Generally, in North American middle-class culture:

- About 21 feet is where we make it clear who we are going to approach or talk to. It is the "first contact" distance. This is also the distance of the famous Tueller drill. An attacker can cover 21 feet faster than most officers can draw and aim a weapon. Coincidence?
- About six feet is where we like to be standing with strangers. It is very close to the "critical distance line." The stranger, if he becomes a threat, must take a step to attack, giving you a little bit of time.
- Four feet or a little less is where we like to talk socially. Some people forget who is a stranger once the talking starts and move closer. Predators who rely on charm to access victims use this tendency.
- About eighteen inches is the intimate distance, how close you like to be when talking to your closest friends. Action being faster than reaction, at this distance it is extraordinarily difficult to stop an unexpected assault.

Proxemics is the study of manipulating these distances.

Couple of caveats: Different societies have different ideas of appropriate distances. Hispanic and Arabic cultures both interact much closer than folks from North America are used to. Another point is that these distances are ingrained and you have an emotional reaction to them. That means that when you work with a culture with a different idea of intimate distance, their "friendly" may be your "creepy." You must adjust.

These distances are measured front to front. People frequently sit with strangers at their sides or behind them (think concerts and sports stadiums) at ranges that would be completely unacceptable face to face. Watch how people stand in an elevator to manage this emotional problem of proximity.

> "S" had been working in Iraq for a while, but he'd never really gotten use to the cultural norms, like men holding hands or kissing cheeks. He was very uncomfortable with how close Iraqis stand when talking. He had some business to do with Haider. Haider liked S, so he took a step closer so he could comfortably put an arm over S's shoulder. S took a step back. Haider stepped closer. S took a step back.
>
> They somehow got the work done, but to an outside observer, it looked like Haider had been chasing S all over the office.

You use proxemics to manipulate your comfort, the threat's comfort, and your safety. Distance is time, and the farther away you are, the safer you are from sudden attack. Twenty-one feet eliminates the sucker punch and gives you plenty of time to put more distance if the threat reaches for a weapon. Safety is always a factor, but it is not the only factor.

You will have a certain comfort level with each person you encounter. That comfort level will show in your preferred distance. That's instinctive. You must be aware that sometimes your instincts are wrong. If you notice yourself moving closer because of a fascinating conversation in a place and time and with a stranger that would normally have you on alert, take a step back. You may be being suckered in.

Safety and comfort are covered. Now on to the threat.

Depending on your purpose, proxemics can be used to either make a potential adversary comfortable or uncomfortable. If you want the other guy to relax, give him distance. Don't crowd. If you are listening to the other guy's problems, it may be appropriate to move closer as the emotional content transitions from outward-directed and angry to inward-directed (guilt, self-pity, or sorrow). If you close unobtrusively and non-threateningly, the other guy will often perceive your proximity as a measure of your friendship.

The emotional brain is stupid (hence easily deceived): "I only let my bestest friends get that close. You're that close? You must be my bestest friend."

You can often get very close by angling. Instead of being directly in front of a potential threat or someone you are trying to calm down, be a little to the side or just off his shoulder. Standing comfortably, like buddies, shoulder-to-shoulder.

The advantage is that as the threat opens up, you can help deal with core issues, settle problems, and prevent violence. There are two disadvantages, however. If it does go bad for some reason, it takes a lot of skill to defend yourself at close range. Second, you may end up with a sloppy, occasionally violent and dangerous drunk who thinks you are his best friend and follows you around like a puppy dog. In some ways that could be worse.

You can also use proxemics to intimidate. This isn't for everybody. For example, Rory who is an infighter by nature and training, routinely steps into intimate distance with violent felons. Most immediately take a step back, which establishes dominance, allows them to skip the verbal sparring, and gets right to solving the issue. The ones who don't instinctively step back are usually infighters as well, in which case there is almost always a mutual respect. But not everyone can pull that off. For example Lawrence, primarily a striker, is more comfortable working at a slightly longer range.

Throughout this book some of you will have a tendency to say, "Oh, yeah. I can fake that. I can do the tough guy vibe or just step into his distance." Don't. Especially here. DO NOT BLUFF that you can go toe-to-toe at biting range. You will be tested and if you react in the slightest bit wrong, you will be mauled and eaten alive.

Crossing lines, say going from stranger to social distance, causes an emotional response in the other person, and usually causes him to react. He has to decide: "Does this guy think we're friends?" "Are we friends?" "Is this guy trying to get into striking range?" "If I back up, will I look like a chicken?"

The power, no matter what he decides, is that he is reacting to you. When someone crosses your lines, you will have the same emotional reactions and the same thoughts.

Practicing positioning is just a matter of reading terrain. When you enter a space, look for avenues of approach and exits, places where you can stand or sit where you can see as much as possible. Identify what would qualify as:

- An obstacle (would slow down a someone trying to get to you or chase you if you leave).
- Cover (would stop a bullet).
- Concealment (not much in the way of physical protection, but you could hide behind it).

Pay special attention to reflections and shadows. With practice, they can cancel out many of the blind spots around you so that you can watch areas without being noticed. Between looking and listening, you should be tough to catch off guard.

Proxemics is harder to practice safely. You will creep people out if you are constantly trying to violate intimate distance just to gauge a reaction. Still, take a seat at a mall or public place and start noticing the correlation of distances between people and the depth of their relationship. Once you become good at it, you are likely to notice some things, like who has started secretly dating, long before your friends or coworkers do.

Display of Force Option

The highest level of pure presence is to give an unmistakable signal that you are willing to go much higher on the force continuum. It raises the stakes and gives the threat one last chance to choose another way.

"Steve," I slid the report back to him, "What the hell did you do?"

Steve was chuckling. "The guy didn't want to come out of his cell, said he'd fight. I didn't want to fight, so I got the Taser and gave him a Taser class."

"You gave him a class?"

"Yeah, I said 'This is an advanced Taser X26' and I sparked it so he could see it arc. Then I said, 'It's 50,000 volts but almost no amps, so it hurts like hell but it won't injure you. See, I pull the trigger and these two darts shoot out, like needles, but they're barbed, sort of like fish hooks. The current runs between the two needles. It hurts a lot and you can't move while the Taser is cycling. People think they'll pee in their pants but no one has yet. Oh, and it runs for five seconds. That can seem like a really long time."

"You gave an inmate a class?"

"Yep, and he decided he really didn't want to fight any more."

Displaying a force option is a potentially high-risk tactic. Courts have ruled that for an officer to threaten a higher level of force than he would be authorized to use IS excessive force. What this means for civilians is that if you draw a gun and could not justify lethal force, you have just committed a crime. If you pull a knife or a gun, even with the intent to prevent things from getting violent, you MUST be able to articulate why the threat had the intent, means, and opportunity to present a lethal threat. And you must be able to state why you had no other option. I.M.O.P. all apply.

There is another safety issue with displaying a force option. Once again, you cannot bluff. If you pull a knife or a gun, or simply raise your fist and threaten, and it does not work, you will have to use what you have threatened. Otherwise, the weapon will be taken away from you and used against you.

This issue is really critical and bears repeating: **If displaying a force option fails to intimidate, you will almost certainly be forced to use it.**

Force options can enter into presence in four basic ways:

1. The presence of a weapon can be implied.
2. The weapon can be displayed.
3. The weapon can be brandished.
4. The weapon can be used to threaten.

Most people who carry a concealed weapon check it from time to time. The checking gesture is one of the things you look for and can be as simple as squeezing your weapon-side elbow against your waist to make sure the holster hasn't shifted or sliding a thumb under your jacket.

If the threat is paying attention, this same type of gesture can imply that you have a weapon. Is there any advantage to the implication? It depends. If the threat has already decided to use force no matter what, he now knows a little more about what he has to accomplish first. Namely, neutralize you and take control of your weapon. You have just raised the stakes.

If, however, the threat is uncertain, the presence of a potential weapon may make him change his mind. Using violence to achieve an end, for the predator, is a pretty cold-blooded risk/rewards calculation. The presence of a weapon vastly raises the risks to the predator. He *may* decide it's not worth it.

It works less well with social violence, and that goes both ways. In a developing monkey dance, there is no place in the steps for a weapon. Unless you consciously break the cycle you don't play the dance, the dance plays you. Consequently, someone caught up in the monkey dance may believe that you will not use the weapon you've displayed. Thinking you won't violate the steps and consequently push the situation, you may very well wind up with a "What are you going to do, shoot us?" scenario. Those tend to end badly.

On January 27, 2005, actress Nicole duFresne was robbed at gunpoint by 19-year-old Rudy Fleming who stole her friend's purse and pistol-whipped her fiancé. What was supposed to be a simple property crime turned tragic when the 28-year-old actress confronted the teenaged robber. She became furious, shoved Fleming, and snapped, "What are you going to do, shoot us?" She died shortly thereafter in her fiancé's arms.

If you are caught in the dance, especially if you mistake predatory violence for social violence, you might disregard the gun as well. We know, we know. Sitting in the comfort of your living room, reading this book, you know you are a logical sensible person. So let's do a thought experiment. You are down at a local restaurant eating with some friends. A couple of the guys have had a beer or two. One of them pulls out his new gun and points it at you. What do you do?

What do you do?

If your absolute first answer wasn't to run like hell, do not be so sure that you would do the reasonable thing. If the thoughts that ran through your head included wondering if the weapon was loaded or which one of your friends had it or how your friends know better, you might well start thinking—trying to engineer a social response—in real life. The monkey brain is deep and powerful. And sneaky.

Displaying the weapon is making sure that the threat knows the weapon is in play. It is not a hint to his subconscious or a subtle change in the flavor of the encounter. It is a message. Whether deliberately showing the holstered weapon or drawing it, deliberate displaying a weapon is very serious. It will likely force the threat to make a decision, either to back down or to attack immediately. Threats, being people, he will probably think about it for a second:

- A predator will do the math, which may include a guess about how fast you can draw.
- A social violence threat may ponder the consequences to his reputation. Backing down from a weapon, in most circles, is considered common sense. It is a face-saving exit. But that's not universal.

If you display a weapon, you are forcing the decision. You have to be ready to act immediately if attacked. At the same time, don't feel you have to do something yourself if nothing happens for a second. In a situation where weapons are out, nothing happening is good. If you don't need to move, wait. Calmly.

Brandishing a weapon is a step beyond this and, generally, is stupid. Waving a gun or knife around to look dangerous or get someone to take you seriously marks you as an amateur, an insecure child. It doesn't make you less dangerous—stupid people with knives are dangerous, too. What it does do is send the signal that others may have to defend themselves; that you are not mature enough to be reasoned with. That means that it justifies massive force to be used against you.

Threatening with a weapon—aiming the gun, raising the club, pointing the knife within striking range at the stomach—is the last step before applying overwhelming force. It should, at this point, not even be considered presence. You are actually in the act of killing. If the threat immediately and unequivocally stops, he may save his own life.

It is critical to think of it this way because there is no half-assed way to do it. You can't change your mind and say, "Just joking." If you do, the threat knows you don't have the guts to use the weapon you are relying on; the witnesses know that you are unstable and dangerous and need to go to prison.

Displaying a force option can be very, very effective. It can also backfire with spectacularly disastrous results. Weigh your options carefully. Remember that any display of a weapon will remove the advantage of surprise if you later need to use the weapon.

Level 1 Conclusion

From mystical to practical, presence is one of the major factors in force incidents. Some people stop fights just by being there. Some start fights. Some people are marked as victims, some as predators. All by presence.

Presence doesn't exist separately from the rest of the force options. When it works on its own, that's perfect. No one gets hurt; there are no lawsuits or paperwork. It augments every other level as well. Stern commands from an authoritarian demeanor work better than the exact same words spoken by a squeaky-voiced teenager. Appeals to reason sound more believable coming from a priest than a psych patient. Scolding works better from a mother figure than a cop.

A joint lock snapped on with authority works better than one applied hesitantly. Someone fist-fighting or using a club who looks like he knows what he is doing makes the adversary more cautious about fighting at all and changes his focus from victimizing to not becoming a victim.

Even at the lethal-force level, a .45 pointed at your head where you can see the bullet at the bottom of the barrel and it looks like a freight train coming at your eyes gets a faster response than an air rifle. A team in black armor working together is more intimidating and much more effective than a bunch of sloppy individuals.

Remember that even at high-end uses of force, you are fighting a mind, not (or perhaps in addition to) a body. Unless the brainstem or upper spine is damaged or every long bone in the body is broken, a threat could *physically* keep fighting. Bad guys (or good guys or even armies for that matter) are not beaten. They give up.

A powerful presence makes it easier for the threat to give up.

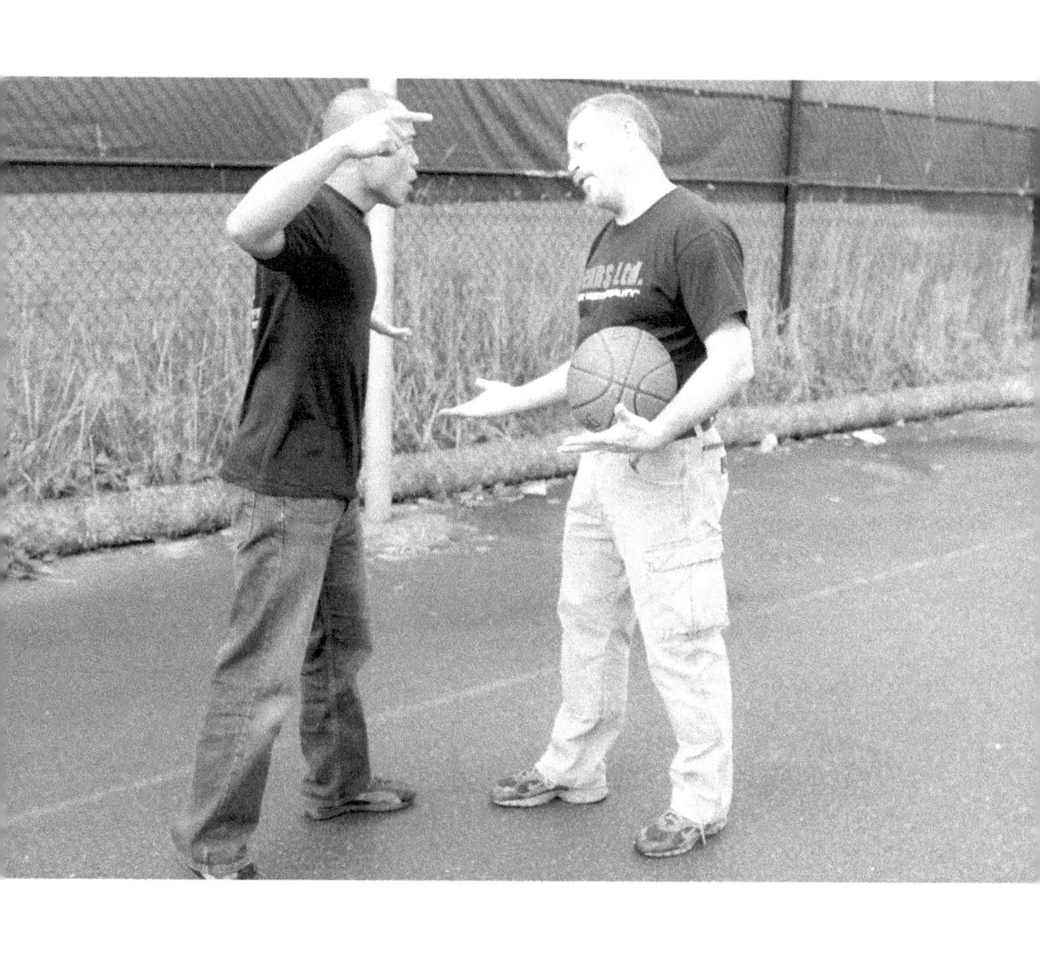

LEVEL 2—VOICE

The inmate was about 6'4" 240 pounds of muscle with a short Mohawk and USMC tattooed on his neck.* He had just come out of our Psych ward and fought three officers on the way. He had been placed in an observation cell. We had just got word that he was to be removed to another facility. He didn't want to go. He wanted to fight.

It's not my area, but they call me. He is in the cell, slamming the Lexan with his fist and elbow, making the walls echo. Medical staff wants him moved to another facility. This means that officers will have to enter the cell, take him down, cuff him, and carry him to a transport vehicle.

So I wander down to the dorm where the sergeant in charge of the area is making the entry plan and a rookie deputy is running around getting belly chains and leg irons. I pull up a chair across from the Lexan door, sit down and get comfortable. First rule: If no one is getting hurt, there is no reason to rush. It's not a macho game—whether I could or not, I have no business going into the cell in some kind of contest. I'll wait, stack everything I can to my advantage and go in fast when the time is right.

The guy is screaming, spit flying out his mouth, slamming his fist again and again into the door, eyes locked on mine. Understand that this is calm for me. There are huge subconscious things going on with dominance and aggression that give most people an adrenaline surge when threatened even if there is no real danger. If you've ever gotten worked up over a phone call or an internet flame war, you know what I mean. For whatever reason, non-standard emotional wiring or experience, I don't get excited.

I'm sitting there, legs crossed, leaning back, hands behind my head and say, "What happened today?"

* I was pretty sure Marine regulation prohibited visible tats, so it was likely a fake. Lots of criminals find an advantage in claiming elite military experience.

"I lost it!" He screamed, "I fuckin' WENT OFF! I need some fucking HELP! MENTAL HELP!"

"That's pretty clear," I said, "Why'd you lose it today?"

He kept screaming, but he was puzzled. The way his world works is this: You get loud and angry, the other person gets loud and angry and then you get violent before he does.

I wasn't working by his rules.

At this point I could feel a palpable rage. I'd been able to smell the adrenaline from the rookie, but this was different. There were waves of rage coming off the inmate, not just rage at me but rage at himself, pure human anger. I decided not to work with the anger.

As he was talking about his breakdown and making threats, I said, "You did good. You did good for a long time. I know you don't like being in a dorm around people but you did it and you did well for a long time. No one can ever take that away from you. You did well and I'm proud of you."

He paused for a second and I said, "It's time for you to go. Will you let me put handcuffs on you?"

He said "yes." He even said "thank you."

Realistically, communication does not exist on a force continuum. Force exists on a communication continuum. Each level of force is simply a more emphatic way to say "No!" We spend more time in this book on physical force because the stakes are higher. You can handle many situations with a kind word. But not a knife coming at your belly.

Before we can begin with the tactics, there are some fundamentals of communication that need to be addressed:

- Range and Style.
- The Players.
- Rate, Tone, Pitch, and Volume (RTPV).

Range and Style

The verbal level is more complex than all of the other levels combined. We are humans; we are communicating creatures. We talk and gesture so much in so many different ways that no single book could cover them all. Much less a chapter.

With regard to preventing violence, verbal skills can range from sweet reason to shouting nonsense while foaming at the mouth (chewing Alka-Seltzer makes a very convincing rabid foam). Logic has its place. So does screaming. Whispering sometimes engages interest when nothing else will. The tactics you might use can range from asking to ordering to commanding to pleading to hinting to confusing.

You will also have a personal style. Some of it will not be under your control. For example, if you have a high-pitched voice, you will have a very difficult time calming people down. Being small is no bar to taking command, but being shy or awkward (or showing the body language that implies shyness) will cancel out your voice no matter how authoritative it is. This is because when your voice sends one signal and your body language sends another, people will assume (quite rightly in the vast majority of instances) that the body language is the truth and the words are a lie.

What this all means is that you already have a personal style of communication. Make sure that your style is congruent with other factors—like the image that you want to project, your mannerisms, and your appearance. If you find that people often dismiss what you have to say, if you are frequently misunderstood, or if you are easily ignored or even ridiculed, your verbal style is almost certainly out of synch with your appearance and presentation.

Unlike higher levels of force, presence and verbal are two integral aspects of your everyday life. It is not just about self-defense. These are things in which you can develop skills. Once you have those skills, every aspect of your life will improve. So, how do you get better at using voice? Here are a few exercises:

- Have a friend describe your voice. Record your own voice and listen to it. Pay special attention to the RTPV (Rate, Tone, Pitch, and Volume). What do you think of that voice?
- Turn off the sound and watch a video of yourself. Look at the characteristics described in the chapter in Level 1 on presence. Does your body language go with that voice?

- Record yourself in normal conversation and, if you can, in stressful conversations, and with different people. Do you get nervous when you talk to your boss? How does it show in your voice? Do you turn into a babbling idiot when talking to members of the opposite sex? What do you sound like on the recording?
- Analyze the voices you hear. Generally, how does each person sound? Cool? Calm? Logical? Strong? Shy? Hesitant? Is what you hear from your own voice what you want to project?
- Watch movies. Older movies are better for this. Ignore the soundtrack, the special effects, and the lighting. Look for those moments when the communication is crystal clear and believable—when the command is a command, when the sympathetic noise really works. Don't get caught by the movie; bad acting can be overcome by a solid script, where everyone sounds as if they are believable. When everything really comes together, ascertain what combination of voice and expression made the line work.
- Then reverse it. Look at the times in the movie when a character says something that just falls flat. Dissect why it fell flat.

The Players

No matter what levels of force you need, the players stay the same. It is critical to be able to read the players.

The threat dictates the situation. You must understand the problem before you can choose a solution. A charm predator is one thing. A drunk wanting to show off for a girl is an entirely different problem. You must learn to read threats and threat dynamics.

We cannot emphasize enough that everything hinges on this:

- Your goal (Escape? Prevail? Get help? Draw attention?)
- Your strategy (Run? Talk? Hide? Fight?)
- Your tactics (Scream or reason? Strike or lock?)
- Your involvement (Is this *your* problem?)

Threat dynamics will be not just influenced, but *dictated* by the problem. You do not get to choose the problem. You do not get to deal with the things your training is good for and skip the rest. **The problem chooses you. You must adapt.**

Part of understanding the threat is listening, a concept that is covered in the section titled "Listening" later in the book. Another part is monitoring. Whatever you choose to do, pay attention to make sure it is actually working. You may have a wonderful plan, but as the old adage goes, few plans survive contact with the enemy. The other guy has plans too.

> Long ago and far away, he had a small group of officers with extra training who were supposed to talk down violent inmates who had made weapons and barricaded themselves in cells. The reasoning was that a person talking is far cheaper than calling out a team.
>
> One of the newer members of the team was intelligent and very personable. Loved to chat. Did really well in classes and had almost a zero percent success rate in real incidents. The officer had never really understood that Crisis Negotiation Teams (CNT) are not really about talking people down as much as they are about listening people down. As long as the officer was talking, she felt that everything was going well.
>
> The officer also seemed to be completely unaware that she had never talked a single inmate into surrendering. The tactical team had to fight every last one she worked on.

You, of course, are the first part of the equation. Much of what you need to think about is covered under the section "Range and Style," earlier in this book. How do you handle this situation? How do you present yourself?

You will also have a role to play. If it is a predatory assault, the threat has already assigned you the role of victim. If it is a dominance display ("You lookin' at my woman?"), you have been assigned the role of rival. Before the assault during the verbal stage, you may be able to pick your own role. By the time the threat becomes physical, it is too late.

In the opening example, the inmate wanted the catharsis of a fight. He wanted to hurt and be hurt. He didn't want to fight one officer because he knew he was going to lose and wanted to lose with what he saw as honor. He would have preferred to fight five or six or ten officers, so he played his script and got angry and loud. He expected Rory to play the other half of his script. To get angry or indignant and rush to call a bunch of officers in for an epic fight would have led nowhere. Rory didn't.

Staying on a script is subconscious. When the script changes, when you don't play your role, the other guy has to think. If the conflict is based on anger, getting the adversary to think can lower his level of tension. With a predator who is deciding to use violence for logical ends, you want him worried, concerned that there are risks of which he is not aware.

The role you choose can be an "end run" around your personal style. Role-playing, even in a real situation, can be effective. How would a drill sergeant handle this? How would a chaplain? You automatically recognize that those are two very different but very effective communication paradigms.

Caution! DO NOT cast yourself in the Billy Bad-Ass role:

- It creates more problems than it solves, especially with witnesses.
- There is a huge price if your bluff gets called. And it frequently will.

Criminals have much more experience bluffing citizens than citizens have bluffing criminals.

The third player in any use of force is the witness or witnesses. When and if the police show up, when and if you are standing in court, the witnesses will be critical to how your act was perceived.

Neither of us is a very emotional fighter, which is good. But even if we did get angry, we would do our best not to show it. Witnesses need to see a professional reluctantly but competently doing what needs to be done. Any abusive language or profanity or threats or even yelling puts that image at risk. Any words or tone that you use before or even during a confrontation can be remembered and will be used to reinforce or to undermine your claim of self-defense. Fear is okay. Showing anger always hurts you.

Legally and ethically, your motivation matters. You shoot someone to stop him from killing a child and you are a hero. You shoot someone because you thought he was an ass, you're a criminal—despite the fact that a guy trying to kill a child is an ass.

Rate, Tone, Pitch, and Volume (RTPV)

The third über-fundamental is RTPV, the rate, tone, pitch, and volume of your voice. This is how people read your emotion, your intent, and your commitment.

Rate and volume are indicators of intensity. The more excited someone is, whether anger or fear or even love—ever watch two teenage girls trying to whisper about romance?—the louder they tend to be. And the faster they talk.

Tone and pitch indicate the quality of emotion. Tone can be difficult to define in a meaningful way, but take the example of a flute and piano both playing the same note (pitch) at the same volume. They still sound different. That difference is the tone. Or maybe the timbre. Whatever. With humans, it is easier—anger sounds different than fear. And different angers have different tones—icy, hissing contempt ("What are *you* doing here?"), or outrage, ("Knock it off!") to name a few. There is something in the tone that even reads as sincerity or follow-through. For example, the guy who is angry and will act on it sounds different than the guy who is really angry but is afraid and will back down. Reading these nuances takes practice, but doing so is very valuable.

Pitch shows fear. Specifically, it shows that the stress hormones have hit the system. People become high-pitched and squeaky under stress, which can be funny...except you might not want funny when talking someone down. This is why having a low-pitched voice is an asset in calming others. It projects a lack of fear, and a lack of fear *is* safety. A high-pitched voice, on the other hand, makes it almost impossible to successfully work with people in crisis. Subconsciously, it is read as fear, and humans, like all primates, find fear contagious.

Always monitor the potential adversary's RTPV. Especially look for changes. If pitch goes up, so has adrenaline. You just moved one step closer to action. If the tone switches from injured to angry, the other guy has just decided on whom to vent his frustration. If rate goes up, the threat is becoming more excited and the situation could break soon, for good or bad. Same with volume.

Control your RTPV as well. These are the elements underlying your speech that indicate to the adversary who you are. Words are merely tricks, in a way. The other guy will decide whether your words can be trusted based on your RTPV and your demeanor. In other words, the threat will not respond to your words so much as he will respond to YOU.

> One RTPV trick: When I get called to deal with agitated bad guys, I initially match their level of intensity. If they are loud and screaming, then I scream too, but just for a second. The first word a touch louder than the threat, and then I drop the rate and volume: "HEY! Hey! Hey."
>
> It is remarkably reliable how the threat will then slow down and quiet down to match me. Sometimes it takes a few repeats. Note that this is volume and rate only. I want the pitch low, showing no fear and offering safety, and the tone is neutral—not angry, fearful or, especially, judgmental.

Listening

> "A wise old owl sat in an oak. The more he saw, the less he spoke. The less he spoke, the more he heard. Why aren't we like that wise old bird?"—A poem done in cross-stitch that used to hang on Rory's mom's kitchen wall.
>
> "A man has two ears and only one mouth so he should listen twice as much as he speaks."—No idea who said this first.
>
> "I don't know that I've ever changed anyone's mind by arguing, but I have changed some by listening."—Rory.

It is amazing how smart and caring people think you are when you keep your mouth shut. People like to talk, and talks often become little ego battles. He said something, which made you think of something else and you cannot wait to tell the story, and then she cuts in with a snide comment and you are afraid the subject will move along before you get to tell your story. Most of the time, in most people's heads, any given conversation is all about them. Not that other people are talking about us. Oh no. We want to talk about us. We want to hear our own voices and tell our stories.

And all the time, everyone is playing this game. It becomes amazing how much talking and how little communicating actually happens. We recognize, at some level, that no one is really listening. Few of us realize that we aren't really listening either.

And in this mess comes a huge opportunity. If you can truly listen, you become some kind of mythical half-human, half-god that people flock to. We are not overstating it. People love to talk, so they talk. But they love to be listened to, to get attention, to think that they are reaching someone—and this aspect is not in their control. It is rare, and makes them feel good. When they come across people who listen well, they spend time with that person. They believe, absolutely, that this quiet, thoughtful, interested person is incredibly smart and compassionate. Sometimes they tell others.

That is the touchy feely side of listening. It has a definite value. Here's the killer tactical side: listening is intelligence gathering. What people say, how they choose to say it, the subjects they avoid and the ones they can't let go, what makes them uncomfortable, the things they lie about all tell you who they are and what they believe. They give you the understanding, which gives you the tools to decide whether or not bad things will happen.

Listening is intelligence gathering; every time you open your mouth, you give some of this away.

I'm not proud of this one. When an inmate threatens suicide, he or she is placed on "suicide watch." All of their items, including clothing, is taken. The inmate is placed in a bare cell. We take the clothing because truly suicidal people can get very ingenious with hanging themselves. We replace it with a paper suit (in the old days) or a quilted, untearable smock.

When I came on shift, this particular inmate had given up everything but her underwear. I was ordered to fix that. Both because it was an order and for the safety of the inmate, I had no choice—she was going to give up her drawers. By force if necessary. I absolutely did not want to write a report about a group of mostly male officers stripping the underwear off a female inmate. I was willing to push as far as I could to prevent a use of force.

She was tearful, angry, only recently arrested and still high. I talked to her for most of an hour and got nowhere. I then got one of our female officers, C to talk to her. C gave it a heroic effort, but after an hour still nothing. I had, however, heard what I needed to hear. I took C aside and said, "I'm about to say something really brutal and then leave. When I go, you play good cop and beg her to give you her stuff. Got it?"

The inmate had mentioned that she had been a victim of sexual violence. That probably contributed a huge amount to this whole scenario. I got loud and faked a lot of anger, told her that I had had it and this had gone on long enough. That she wasn't going to waste our time and jerk us around anymore. That I was going to get the five biggest officers and we were going to go in there, throw her down and tear her underwear off. I stomped off.

C had the underwear out in less than a minute.

I shouldn't feel guilty about this. I deliberately invoked fear in a fragile person, but only to prevent actually using force, which might have injured her as well as triggering the exact same flashbacks as my words. I used everything that she told C (the inmate didn't know that I was out of sight, still listening): the fact of her sexual assault, I even "accidentally" said that the officers I was going to get were the same ethnicity as her attacker.

Was that necessary? It was a lot of pressure, a lot of leverage. It worked. But did I have to go that far? I can't know. If I had used any less and it had failed, we would have been back at square one with the force issue. I do believe that using force would have been worse. I'd do the same thing again.

The point, though, all internal ethical issues aside, is that listening gave me what I needed to avoid force when talking had failed.

Active listening is a skill widely taught in colleges and police academies. It is incredibly simple. It is effective. It helps with everything from dealing with violent offenders to getting along with your significant other. There is no downside to this skill, yet most people do not use it, because it is too important to feel special and the special one is the talker, not the listener. Everyone knows that. Sure.

The basics of active listening are:

- To pay attention. Look at the person talking. Let them see you looking at them. Do not glance at the clock or your watch. Do not start typing on your keyboard, texting on your cell phone, or looking out the window.
- To really, really pay attention. Shut down your own mind. Just listen. In most conversations, person A says something and half way through the sentence, person B has decided what is about to be said, has formulated a reply, and is mentally rehearsing lines. From that point on, person B is not listening. Real communication has already stopped. Listen. Listen all the way through. Then pause and think about it. A pause before answering can also work as a "pattern interrupt." Because you are obviously thinking and listening, the other person must slow down to figure out what is going on and should not count on his own mental scripts. Conversations tend to be deeper and more useful if both people are thinking, actually fully engaged.
- To ask open-ended questions. Remember that this is intelligence gathering. You want to ask questions that cannot be answered with one word. "Did you have a good time Friday?" is closed. "What happened Friday?" is open. The latter encourages a story. You don't just learn from the narrative of events. You also learn about the other person by what he or she emphasizes or leaves out, what makes them excited or subdued.
- To pay attention to the emotion and demeanor as well. When the words say one thing and the emotion says another, bet on emotion for true motive. It can also be a clue when you paraphrase. For that matter, pay attention to your own emotions.

Sometimes they are hints, subtleties your subconscious noticed that have not yet made it to your conscious brain.

- To use feedback/paraphrasing/reflecting. It has a bunch of names. The essence is this: Double-check your understanding. "Let me see if I got this. You were just minding your own business when..." It is good to clear up any miscommunication early. This is also the time to point out body language or incongruities that make you doubt the words (if that is tactically appropriate. Otherwise, it is just a data point). For example, "Dude, you say you're over your ex but every time her name comes up you start grinding your teeth." You can get huge amounts of information when people try to clarify—especially when they are trying to explain away obvious emotion while trying to seem calm.

> If you ask, "What happened between you and Cecilia last night?" and your friend answers: "I shouldn't tell you this, I promised Cecilia I'd keep it quiet but..."
>
> Cecilia's story isn't the only information here. The fact that your friend seems eager to give up secrets may be far more valuable information, especially if you expected him to keep any of your confidences.

Active listening is something you can practice every day. It is a discipline, very much like sitting meditation. You become comfortable and you listen, totally focused. The only difference is that you are focused on another person and might just make his or her day. The same as meditation, when a distraction intrudes, you acknowledge it and return to your focus, this other person.

Feedback is the hardest to practice because it is the one that can sound stilted and gimmicky. Just practice anyway. You will find that feedback follows easily if you have been really listening. If you let yourself get caught up in the story, the paraphrasing will become very natural. "Oh my god! Are you serious? You told the boss to..."

Practice active listening with colleagues and peers. But practice with children, too. The little nippers see things that adults miss. And seniors have seen things that most of us never will. Listening to their memories is good for your soul and good for theirs as well. Really listen to strangers.

There is one downside. People don't get listened to enough, and some can become really attached to you. Basically, some will follow you around like puppies. If you find that annoying, you will have to be able to set very clear boundaries.

Strategic Verbal De-escalation

It's easy to say "talking people down" but you must understand that de-escalation can require very different tactics, depending on the characteristics of each encounter. De-escalating in front of an audience has many more options than de-escalating when you are alone with a threat. De-escalating a process predator (a rapist or thrill killer) is a completely different situation than talking your way out of a barroom brawl.

In all verbal self-defense, you are working directly on the threat's mind. Not always on the same aspect of his mind, however. Largely, you will be working with emotion, the social context, or the threat's equation of risks and benefits.

Changing the Emotion

Anger and fear are the primary emotional reasons that a conflict might escalate to violence. Not always. The predatory violence of a professional criminal can be completely devoid of emotion. When the violence is emotional, however, you can count on anger and fear.

Fear is the easiest in a self-defense context. If the threat is afraid of you, it probably is not self-defense and you can just let the guy leave. There are exceptions. The mentally ill and people on drugs, particularly stimulants and hallucinogens, can be quite dangerous when they are panicky. If you turn the tables in an assault and begin to win, your adversary can panic into a thrashing bundle that becomes very dangerous. Lastly, if the other guy leaves while still afraid but needs some kind of closure or feels humiliated, he may return with enough firepower (or friends) to overcome his fear.

Remember that the lower levels on the force scale are in play before things get physical. In this sense, when dealing with fear, you are talking down an agitated *potential* threat.

Generally, to ease fear you lower stimulation levels and remove dangers. That means low, slow, quiet voices. Only one person talking. Dim lights help, as does turning off the radio or TV or anything that might increase noise, light, or movement. These actions do not include closing doors or even windows, because doing so will make it appear that you are cutting off avenues of retreat. No sudden movement. Do not touch the threat unless it seems necessary. Low-level agitation may ease with a hug from a friend. Animal panic may explode if the person is really afraid. If you are going to touch the person, tell him what you are going to do first. Short words, clear sentences.

The inmate had stripped naked. He had banged his head against the door for a while and then started chewing on his tongue. Now he was howling and spitting blood at the window. Big red flag. Danger, Will Robinson! We call this excited delirium. They sometimes break handcuffs or throw four times their weight in officers around or fight until their heart gives out and then die. Fighting an Excited Delirium (ED) case rarely ends well.

There are only a few people I would have considered adequate as backup. Clyde was one of them. He waited just out of sight as I opened the cell door.

"Hey. The nurse wants to see you."

The inmate glared. But he didn't approach, which was a good sign.

"She's worried about you. You're a mess." No emotion, just fact. RTPV all mellow.

"I'm going to handcuff you and take you to medical." Not a question or a conversation. Just an observation, like talking about the weather. He didn't flinch or bristle; good signs. It was just like soothing an injured animal.

"I'm going to reach out and touch your left arm. Then I am going to put on a cuff." I moved very slowly, not starting until after I had said everything. No questions, no request for permission. He looked at my hand approaching his arm like it was a snake or an alien.

The first cuff went on. This was familiar to him. This was also the crisis point. If anything was going to set him off, it was going to be contact. If it were contact with the cuff and I only got it on one wrist, well, a handcuff swung like a medieval flail can do a lot of damage. I would be at extremely close range with an Excited Delirium case (I'd been there before. I'd been warned about the superhuman strength, but the superhuman speed was a shock the first time). Clyde might be a couple of seconds hearing something go wrong and getting through the door. A lot can happen in a couple seconds.

"Please turn around. Then I'll put on the other cuff." He complied. "Clyde, could you hand us a blanket?" That gesture may not have penetrated to his conscious mind, but somewhere he took it as care-taking, respectful of his dignity.

Nothing bad happened.

Be aware of what the threat is afraid of or angry about. If you can remove those elements from the equation, you can go a long way toward preventing an escalation to violence. The most common fears that lead to violence are social. If the threat perceives a challenge, he is likely afraid to back down in front of his friends.

Give him a face-saving way out. "Man, if we did fight, you'd probably kick my ass. Let's just skip that step and have a beer."

If you increase the humiliation, you increase the fear of social fallout. "Punk, if you don't want to spend the night in the hospital, walk away." That approach might work. Or it may force the other guy to save face by fighting. Or to hedge his bets by bringing friends or weapons (or both) into the situation. Possibly more importantly, you played Billy Bad-Ass and witnesses will remember that. Proving self-defense will be difficult at best.

To gauge the social stakes, look at the witnesses:

- If the witnesses include (for a young male threat) women, he will be far more afraid of losing face than otherwise. Belittling and challenging is rarely, if ever, a good tactic, but it's guaranteed to backfire here.

- Same with a father or mother in front of their family. If they see you as a threat to their children, they may ramp up the violence well beyond a level you are ready for.
- If the threat is part of an identifiable group (gang colors, guys all wearing the same team jackets), the group will give you clues. If they are watching hungry, he may be their dedicated roper, the guy who picks fights so that everyone can join in. If so, give no hooks (actions the threats can use as an excuse to attack you) and get out through a very public and well-lit place as soon as possible. If his group, however, is looking over like they are embarrassed, he is probably the newbie looking for a reputation. If your cold-conversation skills are good, strike up a conversation with the leader of the group. This exchange does not have to be about the threat. It puts you, socially, out of the newbie's reach. It then becomes up to the leader whether you merit special treatment.
- If you are a member of an identifiable group (e.g., if you have friends with you) and a threat approaches, keep an eye out for his friends. It may be a set-up (very unlikely unless you are a cop, a college athlete, or a gang member), but more likely he is just drunk and stupid. Do not humiliate him because your being with a group increases his internal justifications to get a gun out of his car, but do include your friends in the conversation. A good wing man can step in and completely distract the threat just by starting a conversation about anything except you.
- If there are no witnesses, put yourself on red alert. Social context drives social violence and it usually requires an audience. If there is no audience, especially if the threat has approached you, set your brain for predatory violence. There are very few good reasons for a violent criminal to want to be alone with you. It is not just that, unlike in social violence, the predator is not playing to an audience. He is actively avoiding witnesses. In this case, default to the steps under the section "Changing the Equation" below.

There are two ways to defuse anger and they depend on the type. There is anger, and then there's asshole anger. People get angry, and then they want to hit things. Some assholes become angry, decide they want to hit somebody, and then go fishing for an excuse.

If someone is just balls-to-the-wall enraged, screaming and throwing things, and knocking over tables, there are a few questions you need to ask yourself:

- Is this my problem? Unlike police officers, citizens generally have no duty to get involved. Unless you are an immediate potential victim, a guy throwing a temper tantrum is not your responsibility. There may be cases when you feel differently. If the threat is a friend or relative, you may feel a need to intervene before someone calls the police. If the guy is wrecking your place of business, you should definitely call the cops first, but you may feel a responsibility to talk the guy down for the safety of your other customers.
- Is he mad at me? A guy in a generic rage (dropped his own beer after losing his paycheck gambling and his wife is leaving) is one thing. A guy pissed at you (just figured out that you spilled his beer, you beat him at pool, and his wife is leaving him for you) is something else.
- Do I need to be here? Preclusion is paramount in claims of self-defense, and definitely here. Can I leave? Better the threat break every plate and all the furniture in the house than to injure a person.

De-escalating someone who is mad at you as an individual is challenging. Most people screw it up because they subconsciously shift from trying to eliminate the anger to trying to get an affirmation. Get this: If the guy is screaming, "Get out of my house or I'll kill you!" the best de-escalation is to leave without saying a word. Anger is adrenaline-based and very few men can keep up a good rage for more than half an hour. Women can.

The worst de-escalation is to say something like, "Okay, I'll leave, but I want you to know I'm really sorry and I hope we can be friends again someday." Get it? That's not about the angry guy or the situation. That is an insecure schmuck trying to get someone who is really pissed to tell the schmuck that he is a good person. Don't be a schmuck.

It's natural, because almost everybody feels the need to get the last word in, to "find closure," and to be affirmed in our value as human beings. Natural, but highly inappropriate here. Seriously, if your value as a human being is measured by what a raving, frothing enraged person thinks of you, you probably need help.

A lot of anger-based conflict comes with instructions: "Get out of my face!" "Shut up!" "Get the hell out before I hurt you!" Follow the instructions. And leave. Give angry people time to cool down and remove whatever they are focusing their anger on. If a guy is personally mad at you, it is often best to get someone else to talk to him. The inability to recognize when you are a major part of the problem is dangerous.

When the rage is more impersonal, assuming it is inappropriate to leave, there are a few things to do. Just like with fear, lower the stimulation level. Control your own RTPV. If possible, give time and silence. Anger takes a lot of energy and most people exhaust themselves quickly.

If you are going to talk, don□t be judgmental. DO NOT tell the person what to think, do, or feel. Has someone ordering you to calm down ever worked? It is irritating enough when you're not already furious. If you are going to talk at all, ask a question. Ask a relevant, reasonable question. "Paul, you're clearly pissed. What happened?" Then shut up and listen.

This approach does two things. Talking takes time and time burns off adrenaline. The rage decreases. Second, and possibly most important, it is hard to tell a story or explain things while enraged. People love to talk. Especially about themselves.

There is some danger, especially if a threat is in a drug-fueled rage or other altered state of consciousness, that you may become the focus. It's a risk. One tactic that often works is to say, "No. You weren't mad at me when you came in, but you were already mad. This isn't about me. What happened?" Presented with calmness, sounding like you're willing to help (but not willing to go along with bullshit) works on relatively sane, sober people. Many tactics can work when dealing with altered states of consciousness, but none work with perfect reliability.

Asshole angry is a different matter. These are guys looking to pick a fight. It is a very specific pattern with all the worst elements of whiny entitlement and bully arrogance. The whiny entitlement comes into the situation with the insults. When an asshole calls you a "motherfucker" or a "piece of shit," well, that's free speech. If you return the insult, you're oppressing him and deserve a beating. See the pattern?

> Locally a while back a teenager decided to screw with another driver. For several miles, he boxed the driver in against the rail, speeding up to prevent him from passing, slowing down when the driver tried to slow down. He thought it was great fun, until the other driver pulled a gun.
>
> The kid who was cutting off the driver was getting off on the power of making someone else angry. Drawing a gun was wrong, there will be consequences, but only a moron would be surprised that provoking anger led to—you guessed it—anger.

That's the game of the asshole. When he wants to fight, he may have picked you or just thinks you have potential, so he tries to provoke you into justifying what he wants to do already. It is like fishing. You can think of the provocations as hooks. Understand that he has (possibly subconsciously, but almost certainly consciously) already decided what he wants to do. His pre-assault game is to find an excuse, a justification, something that when he is bragging with his buddies later will make him sound like less of an ass.

> Most of what we are writing in this book is stuff that has worked for us. Some of it I hesitate to recommend. This is one that requires finesse and caution but is extremely powerful: I call people on lies directly. In the environment where I worked, calling someone a liar was an almost guaranteed fight-starter. But I did it, reliably and very successfully.
>
> First off I never said, "You're a liar." Unless the guy asked directly. I usually said, to a specific statement, "That's not true." Or "That's not right." He would freeze for a second and I would explain my reasoning, "If you were diagnosed with paranoia, you wouldn't have come up to talk to me, you wouldn't be standing this close, and your body language would be entirely different." While he was digesting that, I'd kick it back, "You told me that because you wanted to make a point. Let's start with the point, with what you want, and I'll see if I can help with that."
>
> Because the statements were non-judgmental (as much as possible) and calm, my reasoning was out on the table, they could not argue with it (though some

tried). I made it clear that I was willing to help with the underlying problem, if it were reasonable.

This approach worked very well, and many inmates found it easier to talk to me directly and just skip the lying and games. But it's not for everyone...

"I beat up this guy for no reason," does not play well, even in criminal circles. "I beat up this guy because he insulted me," sounds much better.

The asshole game can mimic the early stages of the monkey dance with the hard stare and verbal challenge ("What you lookin' at?"). It can follow all the steps of the monkey dance with the exception that the asshole will strike early, hard, and for damage. He wants to deliver a beating, not establish dominance. He likes giving pain.

Differentiating between an asshole and someone monkey dancing can be easy. There are standard ways to back down from the monkey dance—lowering your eyes and apologizing, changing the subject, and treating the challenges as thoughtful questions. If these fail, if the person pretends to be insulted no matter what you say, be prepared for an asshole. You will see this dynamic in a lot of places, including boardrooms and road rage. If it is up close and personal, the person will be an experienced street fighter.

An asshole without an audience should be treated as a predator. He is, in fact, a low-level process predator who, instead of rape or murder, enjoys beating. If there is an audience, play them to create witnesses. Making statements that the audience can hear helps create witnesses who will be sympathetic to your cause if or when the police arrive or you have to go to court, and can even bring on intervention on your behalf occasionally. Whatever you say, make it low key and make sure that everyone hears it. Do not give up a hook—keep the language clean, don't insult, threaten, or brag—but get some attention.

"You're obviously trying to make me angry. I don't even know you. Leave me alone."

Cockroaches don't like light and assholes don't like witnesses (unless they are roving in packs). When dealing with a pack, it is not something you are likely to talk your way out of unless there is an authority figure nearby. Even a large crowd is not much protection.

A single friend might pull someone back, whether monkey dancing or asshole fishing. But very few people will interfere with a pack. Get out. It will turn into a group monkey dance once you are in the sights. And you will be hurt.

In the aspect of seeking justification for something they have already decided to do, you will see a parallel with some rapists. They have a need to blame the victim.

Changing the Social Context

As previously mentioned, social violence happens in a social context. Generally, disputes arise over status (including "respect"), territory (including symbols), and rule-breaking. Some types mimic the violence of a predatory assault. Others, especially when a group turns on an individual, can be horrific.

Disputes over status rarely escalate to violence, except with young men. It rarely escalates because friends step in and separate the two. This is one of the reasons why an audience is so critical—there are others. An un-witnessed victory is not a victory. Status always occurs within a group. The people you are trying to impress should be present. The group's function, their part of the "social contract," however, is to prevent damage. Separating two fighters (or two almost-maybe-thinking-about-fighting people) is the classic face-saving exit.

Both participants can claim that only the intervention of others prevented an ass kicking and they can now share the same territory without much growling.

There are a number of strategies for de-escalating status violence. You can leave. You can, almost always, simply apologize. You can treat any challenge as a thoughtful question. For example, a response to "What you lookin' at?" might be "Sorry, bro, the brunette cocktail waitress was right over your shoulder. Wasn't staring at you."

Sometimes, you can co-opt a challenger, especially if you are new:

"That's my chair."

"Figures. I'm new here and don't know the players. Fill me in?" It is almost impossible to ask someone to teach you disrespectfully.

You can remove yourself from the society. This is not a physical action, or doesn't need to be anyway. Most status challenges are between young men in the same basic group. The first to get a job or go to college or join the military puts a distance between himself and the rest. It is now expected that his challenges will be in that group. Violence can arise from other reasons, usually asshole reasons, but openly gay men are largely excluded from the monkey dance. Women and children are exempt, except in the minds of some very twisted or confused people. No one likes to monkey dance with the mentally ill because they may not follow the rules and there is little status to be gained. Being an off-duty cop takes you right out of the running. Claiming to be one if you aren't, however, is a crime.

Playing the "older and more mature" game can work as well. Like with all verbals, the game must fit your style and you have to do it sincerely. If you are a jerk deep down, none of this will work for you. If you aren't a jerk, and you're the right age (or appear to be), you can play a wise father figure, "Son, we have no quarrel. I think you want to impress that pretty young thing over there. You want some advice from an older man? Go pay attention to her. Dance, whatever. Don't pay attention to some old stranger like me."

You can also manipulate the audience directly. When a young inmate seeking a rep started to push, Rory would often turn to a well-respected older con and say, "This young man could use some advice about how to get along in the world. You mind having a talk before he gets himself in trouble?"

More generally, loud enough for many to hear, "This isn't a grade-school playground. We aren't children. We aren't going to fight."

You must be careful to avoid humiliating the other guy, but sometimes just ignoring works very well. He begins the first step of the monkey dance, you look at him and go right back to talking to your friends or whatever you were doing. If he escalates, he looks silly. If he approaches, he draws attention. If he does approach with the, "Are you ignoring me?" you can say, "No, I was just busy. Did you have a question?" Or, depending on style, "Yes, I was."

Either of these (the first because of the "have a question" tag line) is off script enough that he will have to think to respond. Getting the other guy to think is half the battle. Remembering to think yourself is more than half the battle; if you are acting on emotion, none of this will work.

The monkey dance and the educational beat-down and other social violence patterns are subtle. They don't take a lot of time or involve vast areas of the participant's lives. Other patterns are more all-encompassing. There are victim personalities. Some children are not only raised with abuse, but groomed to be acquiescent and think that abuse is normal, even love. There are abusive, codependent relationships where the moment of violence or the immediate precursors are just a small part of a larger dynamic.

These are not the kinds of problems that can be solved with techniques. No self-defense class or verbal skills will do more than slow down these train wrecks. What has to happen is deeper, more difficult, and usually fails. The victims MUST do the deep work to change who they are. "Victim" is not just a label; someone is not a victim just because of what happened. When they have been raised and trained to be a victim, victimhood becomes part of their identity. They think, act, and understand as victims. Not merely as people who have been victimized but as people who make it easy for others to prey. They are not just people bad things happen to, but people who live in and seek out the bad things. Is this blaming the victim? No more than saying malnourished children will have predictable health problems later in life.

If you are stuck in one of these destructive patterns, you must change. It will be an immense act of will. It can be done.

Another type of social violence happens when you break a rule. This is especially critical when you are out of your environment. Every place and group of people have unwritten rules. You know the ones where you live, work, and play even if you could not list them. You know how close you can stand to a stranger, what words are not permitted. Whom you greet and whom you ignore.

All groups have these rules and all groups enforce them. In some circles, they are enforced with a raised eyebrow or a "chat" or a memo. In other groups, the rules are physically enforced. If you are a member of a group that uses physical force, this is not news to you. If you come from genteel and educated people in a highly civilized part of the world, this fact may be a shock.

In some parts of the world, breaking social rules are punished with sanctions ranging from a spanking to getting punched in the arm or thwacked on the head, to a beating to being buried alive, to being murdered and mutilated in front of an audience. Those last two, obviously, are not for the benefit of the offender, but to send a message to everyone else.

> In September 1992, shock jock Howard Stern insulted Filipinos on his radio show by saying, "I think they eat their young over there." He was promptly challenged to a duel by Rene Santa Cruz, a DJ at radio station DZXL in Manila (whose employer, Radio Mindanao Network, agreed to pay his expenses to the duel site). This wasn't a publicity stunt, but rather an actual death-threat in keeping with Santa Cruz's cultural upbringing. Stern later apologized. According to the Orlando Sentinel, the Filipino-American Citizens group also sued Stern for $65 million in New York court over the incident.

This is all in the nature of an educational beat-down. When you step into a new group, you don't know what the rules are or how they are enforced. Pay attention. Stay low key. Keep your mouth shut.

This approach is a good rule for business too. Do not challenge anything or make waves, even with the best intentions, until you have been there for a while. Start by asking a lot of good questions, learn the norms of the group, show you are intelligent and have a good attitude. Then make a contribution. There may or may not be good reasons for things running the way that they do, but if you start off all hellfire to make changes right out of the gate you may cause more problems than you are trying to solve. And you will almost certainly piss people off. They may not beat you physically, but ill-will can make you just as miserable in the boardroom as it can in the barroom.

The best verbal defense to an impending educational beat-down is a sincere apology. Not an excuse or an attempt to mitigate responsibility, but an apology.

"I'm sorry, I didn't know. It won't happen again" is acceptable, while "Sorry, but I don't think you should blame me. No one told me I couldn't do that" is not. It's weaseling. The reason apologies work, when they do, is that you have shown that you understand that *you* did wrong, feel bad about it, and won't do it again. Weaseling, trying to evade or attempting to shift blame, is proof that you don't get it. That invites a beat-down.

Apologize, sincerely. Then go someplace where you can make a mistake without bleeding.

Changing the Equation

I'd worked late, but not that late; it was a bit after 6:30 at night. Nevertheless, the garage was nearly deserted. Four cars beside my own were still parked on the third level, none within a dozen feet of my vehicle.

I heard him before I saw him, and something about his gait made me look up. He was tall, almost painfully thin, and dressed in ratty clothing. He didn't quite look like a transient, but not by much. Wasn't wearing an ID badge either; I couldn't imagine that he was a fellow employee. More worrisome, his body language was wrong. He was closing too fast, and his focus was way too intense.

Then one hand strayed toward his waistband.

Blading my body, I prepared to use my laptop bag as an impromptu weapon. And wondered how the hell I'd be able to explain to my boss why I'd broken a company computer. Had I backed it up before leaving? How hard it would it be to get my data back...

"I wonder how long they keep the tapes in those security cams," I mused aloud.

Startled, he glanced up. And stopped advancing.

I quickly climbed into my car and started the engine. He just stood there while I drove away.

Predatory criminals do not work off emotion, if you disregard feelings of power and satisfaction that predators get from raping, murdering, or beating someone. Nor do they give a damn about social status. They care a great deal about not getting caught. The predator wants what you have. He wants to get it in the safest, easiest way possible. That means that he will gather some intelligence on you. All it may take is a glance:

- Isolated place? Check.
- Victim that fits the profile? Check.
- Victim not paying attention? Check.

That's all a robber, serial killer, or rapist may need to know. The question is not whether he can take your stuff. Or do bad things to you. By the time most people grow into full-blown predators, they have had a lot of experience and are pretty confident about their skills. The question is whether or not they can get away with it.

Sometimes it takes more. We've covered this in the 'Victim Interview' section of "Situational Awareness," but will go into a lot more depth here: it is called the victim interview when a criminal approaches a potential target and tries to size him or her up with a conversation. It can be as simple as "Buddy, got a match?" The professional threat will look at how you answer—not at all, terse, or wordy and apologetic. Wordy and apologetic is a good sign that you would be easily dominated.

The pro will look at your attention:

- Looking away—easily dominated.
- Scurrying away—easily dominated but not worth chasing if it will draw attention.
- Turning full on to face him—exposing your underbelly, probably *trained* to be easily dominated. But this impression can be modified by hand and foot position.
- Blading—turning the body so that one side is more toward him and feet are ready to launch—and keeping him in peripheral vision—not worth the trouble.
- Scanning the threat then checks the area—player.

The pro will look at what you do with your hands. If you dig your hands in your pockets looking for matches, you are helpless. If you make a big show of checking all your pockets for a lighter even though you and the threat both damn well know you don't smoke, the threat knows you are a pleaser, not only easy to victimize but likely to "donate" with just a little hint of intimidation. If you keep your hands free and ready, not usually a good choice. If you blade one hip slightly away and check for something under the jacket at the belt line—well, the professional threat knows when he is outmatched.

Communication at this level is much more than just talking. When talking is involved, there are a few points that most people have trouble with. You do not need to say anything. This is not a conversation that you started. Silence is an answer. Will it piss him off? Maybe, but here's the deal: This isn't a monkey dance. A monkey dance will not begin with someone asking you for something. It makes no sense in a domination contest to ask for a favor. If you ignore a predator in an interview, he may try to mimic the monkey dance or call you names, but that is not his intent. His intent is to engage you.

Here is the way this conversation might go:

"Hey, man, you got the time?"

You ignore him.

"What are you? Some kind of stuck-up prick who won't help a brother out? You too good to talk to the poor?"

If he hits your buttons (and he is good at it, this is what he does to get money for drugs and he needs a lot of money to feed his habit every day) you might feel suddenly guilty and say, "Oh, no, nothing like that. I didn't mean to seem rude."

And the threat follows up with, "Man, I was just going to ask if you could help me out with a couple bucks to get home." You guilt button is already hit. You may pay up. If you don't, the threat can repeat step two until you pay up or tell him, assertively, to back off.

This is called "aggressive panhandling" in many jurisdictions. It is somewhere between a shakedown and a con; there is an art to it. It follows the same dynamic as many robberies, so get to know this pattern; it is very similar with many street-level criminals. One of the beauties is that the victim rarely reports a crime and the prosecutor could never make a case stick. The criminal knows there is zero chance of jail. Low benefit, maybe just a couple bucks, but also zero risk. And who knows, the victim may flash a wallet with a couple hundred in it while digging out the two bucks. Then it might be worth it to draw the knife and escalate—if there are no witnesses.

□No□ is a complete sentence. So is "Back off."

The second point is that people talk too much. It is probably not conscious, but criminals very well know the difference between social and asocial violence. If you are talking, trying to explain yourself, the predator knows that you are thinking in terms of social conflict. That means that you are (also subconsciously) expecting a specific script to play out with a specific, predictable outcome. You also believe that violence won't happen unless certain conditions are met, and if violence does happen, it will be mild and the damage likely cosmetic.

If that sounds like too much to think about, don't worry about it. You are not thinking it. This is the way you have been programmed from birth and the way humans have been wired since we roamed the savannah. You have separate programs for dealing with threats from people and danger from lions. These abilities are internal and unconscious. If the threat knows you will treat him like a person but intends to act like a lion, he has a huge advantage.

So just say "No." Or just say, "Back off!" Don't explain yourself. Don't answer questions. Don't debate. Statements like these are boundary-setting, not conversations. If you start talking, you compromise your boundaries.

Once boundaries are set, you will need to defend them. If you say "Back off!" or "Don't touch me!" and the threat closes anyway, you will have to get physical. Remember I.M.O.P.? Closing or touching after these statements shows clear intent. The threat, by closing, is gaining opportunity. His fist, boots, and possible weapons are the means. You must choose an appropriate level of force, but if your boundaries are violated you will need to use force. If you don't, the boundaries were never real to begin with. Worse, your adversary now knows this and will never believe that your no means no. Now you're screwed.

This is paramount, so it warrants repeating—two things people have trouble with are:

- Choosing not to talk at all.
- Keeping it short and harsh when setting boundaries.

Taking your money is a job, like any other. The threat weighs the risks and the benefits. If the benefits far outweigh the risks, the bad guy takes the job. One of the best strategies you have is to make the predator doubt his equation. Just like your equation, the threat's equation is based on the victim, the threat, and witnesses.

You have little chance of casting doubt on the threat himself. He knows what his track record and abilities are when it comes to taking people down. You can, however, cast doubts on his assessment of you. It's all about risk and reward.

For example, if you talk to yourself, loudly and angrily (even better if you talk to someone who is not there) while making gestures and staring around, the threat will have to re-evaluate. Unless you have a Bluetooth in your ear. Crazy people are unpredictable when attacked and tend to carry little money. (This must be congruent with your attire, however. Crazy in a $2,000 silk shirt doesn't sell horribly well.)

If you know how to set boundaries, you raise the risks for the threat.

If there are no real witnesses, you can allude to them anyway. Talking to someone on the cell phone, is a good example: "I'm at Fifth and Hornesby. No, it's pretty quiet. There's just one guy here, he's at the bus stop. I don't know, average I guess. Pockmarked face, green hat, and a jeans jacket..."

You can really work on his paranoia, provided it is early in the interview. Or you can pre-empt the interview by starting it yourself: "Is something going on? That's the second unmarked cop car I've seen cruising by in the last five minutes."

If you can indicate that the environment is going to change soon, such as by talking to yourself, then the threat will have to work fast or not at all. "Dammit. Frank and Jim were supposed to be here ten minutes ago." Successful tactics here either must be real or extremely well-played. If the threat gets any idea that you're bluffing, if he believes you are talking for his benefit instead of out of frustration, it will increase his confidence.

When intervening as a third party, such as trying to break up or prevent a fight or assault, you can add information—"I think I hear sirens." "I saw someone drive by and start punching numbers on a cell. I think it was 911." "Hey, someone called the cops."

Very disturbing, because this tactic works better on criminals is: "Dude, I don't think he's breathing." For someone who is not used to fighting and thinking about the legalities, it would take a while for the significance to sink in. For many violent professional criminals, they spring away. The stakes have gone way up—assault has become manslaughter, may become murder if the threat stays.

Raising the Stakes

Sometimes inmates don't like to be released. Sometimes it is because they have no place to go and it is cold outside. Sometimes because all of their friends are inside. Sometimes because they are afraid to call their parents for a ride home from jail.

I was taking an inmate to release. He was a young man and had made it very clear that he didn't want to be released just yet and thought it should be his choice. As we stepped on the elevator he said, "I bet if I hit you I'd get to stay in jail."

"Technically, no. You'd still leave. Just to the hospital."

"What?"

"Hit an officer, go to the hospital."

"Is that a threat?"

"Oh, no," I sounded apologetic and tried to sound self-effacing. "It's just policy." It wasn't of course. Even under assault, most officers were pretty good about keeping cool.

He looked me up and down as the elevator moved to the ground floor. He couldn't figure it out. I was smaller than him, calm and relaxed, talking about hospitals and cause-and-effect.

I pushed for resolution. I didn't want him to decide not to hit me and then later decide to lash out with the release officer. "Looks like you need to make a decision. I get a paycheck whether you go to the hospital or not. What's it gonna be?"

"I won't be any trouble."

Raising the stakes is a tactic that works at several levels. If you do the math, it is impossible for a small woman to resist a committed attacker. He will be stronger, bigger, and have surprise and a plan on his side. Purely crunching the numbers, the victim does not have a chance.

But victims have won.

Many, many times they have fought their way to safety, or scared off, or incapacitated the threat. So what's going on? The math (size + strength + predator surprise) of what should happen in an assault doesn't match observations from the field.

There is a certain inherent risk in being a predator. The predator does everything he can to minimize the risk, that is his job, but the risk exists. Sometimes the rabbit turns on the fox. Sometimes the cat scratches the dog instead of running. When the eight-pound cat scratches the eighty-pound dog and the dog runs, it is not because the dog couldn't win. It is because the dog decided the price was too high.

Raising the stakes is merely setting the price higher. Sometimes the threat will decide the price of admission is too high to stay in the game. In general, a threat will rarely pick a larger, stronger, alert victim. But that's not the way the game is always played.

Countervailing force can backfire. An article written in the eighties provided a statistic that fighting back against a rapist decreased the chances of rape by around 80 percent and increased the chance of being killed by 13 percent. (Reading statistics is a skill, and this one was unsourced, so it couldn't be analyzed. Nevertheless, it is highly unlikely that 13 percent of rapes turned to murders. That would be an astronomical number, whereas a 13 percent increase from the current murder rate in a rape is a much smaller number.)

At the verbal level of the force continuum, raising the stakes is a tactic that entails letting the threat know that the fight he thinks he is getting may not be the one he will get. It is not the game that Marc MacYoung refers to as "escalato," where each person in the monkey dance throws a little more ego in until they are too committed to leave. Escalato is largely internal; both parties make bigger and bigger threats, but the reason they stay in the game is fear of looking cowardly if they quit. Both parties become too emotionally invested to quit. And unless there is an intervention, someone gets hurt.

Making a big threat is a form of raising the stakes. The threat can scare off the other guy. Maybe. But remember that you are also creating witnesses. If you boldly state that if he does not back down, you are going to kill him, chop him up, and mail his bloody body parts to his wife and children, or rip his head off and piss down his throat, or tear his arm off and beat him to death with it, you won't be able to claim self-defense later. Statements like that allow the other guy to claim self-defense. Legitimately.

Better than a challenge or a threat, you can raise the stakes simply by implying that what you have to fight for is pretty precious. "Partner, I'm on parole and I am not going back to prison for some little fight. Leave me alone." If you are going to prison whether the fight is serious or not, there is no penalty for making it serious. This is the kind of tactic, however, that works better on criminals who understand the words than it does on ordinary civilians.

Or the classic—"Today is a good day to die." It has to be sincere, believable, but only if you are ready to die to make someone pay for what they do to you. That is a level of commitment that most won't want to match.

Raising the stakes can be risky, but it can also keep conflict at the verbal level when the other guy wants to do more.

Tricks and Tactics—Miscellaneous Stuff

There are thousands of little things that help with communication. Everything ties together. After Hostage Negotiator Training (HNT), officers were advised to read books on salesmanship for follow-up reading. It was really the same thing, talking someone down and closing a deal.

Everything works both ways

That applies to both learning and application. If you read about conmen preying on the gullible, you are learning. Your inclination will be to identify with the victim and try to figure out how to see a con and protect yourself. Reverse it. How did the con get the person to trust? What in his tactics can I use to get people, especially potential enemies, to like and trust me? It sounds manipulative, but it is the highest order of strategy to turn an enemy into a friend.

The same thing applies in an application: If you have considered raising the stakes, be alert for the potential threat who tries to raise the stakes with you. It is a sign of his fear. The other guy's fear gives you opportunity.

In Gavin DeBecker's book, *The Gift of Fear*, he lists and describes verbal tactics that a predator uses to talk his way into a victim's good graces—and into striking range. The tactics that he lists there—forced teaming and loan-sharking in particular—are exactly the tactics that work to develop rapport, to keep a criminal from becoming angry, and get the other guy to open up.

Forced teaming

Forced teaming is simply the tactical use of the word *we*. "We don't seem to be getting along. Why do you think that is?" "What should we do about this problem?" Using the word "we" is a way to imply that you and the threat are a team, in this together. Part of the same group. A predator uses the tactic with the intention to betray that trust. You can use it to develop trust and turn a threat into an ally.

Loan-sharking

Loan-sharking is the simple act of small favors. Done by criminals, it creates a feeling of debt and evokes vulnerabilities. Done by people of good heart it is "random acts of kindness and senseless acts of beauty." This is a critical concept, not just for everything in this book but for everything in life. There is no division between "good" tactics and "evil" ones, nothing that criminals use that good guys do not also use. Bad people can and will use anything (charities, civil rights legislation, compliments, etc.) for bad ends. Good people will use the exact same things for good ends.

Co-opting

Co-opting is getting someone on your side before they have decided that you are a rival. It prevents a lot of social violence and it is a key skill when you are on unfamiliar ground. When you do not know the rules of behavior it is easy to unintentionally insult people. The problem is that if you don't know the rules, you also don't know how the rules are enforced. If you come from a society where a social blunder is treated with a sneer or silence, you are probably completely unprepared and will freeze if a mistake is treated with a beating or a blade.

Co-opting requires sincerity, a little curiosity, and humility. It can be as simple as saying, "I'm new here. What are the rules?" It immediately indicates that you won't monkey dance for status. Asking to be taught designates the other as a teacher and acknowledges a higher status. A sincere request to be taught is rarely taken as disrespectful.

As the relationship progresses, be sure to ask about power structures too. It is important to know who is in charge and who works with and against whom.

Congruence

Congruence is having your total message come through with power. You are congruent when your words, RTPV, demeanor, and body language all send the same message. It is received as both sincere and serious. This concept is important because most people do not speak with a lot of congruence most of the time. You should never have to say, "I'm serious." Your body language and tone should say that for you.

Congruence is one of the standards that you evaluate by seeing yourself communicate. Watch yourself on video when you can. Also evaluate good actors, the ones who make you believe a speech. How do they achieve congruence?

Incongruence

Incongruence can be just as useful as congruence provided it is used consciously. Basically, if your words and body language do not match, the adversary will believe your body language. There are a few exceptions. Certain mental illnesses prevent the sufferer from reading expressions. Saying, "I don't want to fight," while rubbing your fist and grinning like a maniac feels like a trap to the threat. It increases doubt.

Non-sequiturs

Sometimes saying something outrageous, something that makes no sense, can freeze an adversary for a second as his brain adjusts. If you realize that de-escalation is not working and that you will have no other choice but to fight, it may also be possible to cause your opponent to make a mental twitch, providing a moment of opportunity to counterattack while he mentally shifts gears. This twitch is brought about by dissonance between what the person expects and what you actually say or do.

A common example is asking a question. While the bad guy is focusing on your words or thinking about an answer, you have a moment in which to run or strike. This may be particularly useful when confronted with multiple assailants. Ask something completely unexpected like, "What time is it?" or something really odd like, "What was Gandhi's batting average?" Cognitive dissonance is powerful. During the opponent's momentary confusion, you will have an opportunity to act.

Similarly, if you believe that you must strike preemptively, you can hit an aggressor while he is talking and it will take him about half a second to mentally switch gears from communicating to fighting. That is a pretty long time in a fight, particularly for a seasoned boxer, martial artist, or street fighter who can throw as many as half a dozen full-power blows in a half-second.

Boundaries

Boundary-setting is critical when dealing with potential threats. Boundaries are especially important when dealing with people who are not overt threats but are in a position of trust—people you are dating, for instance. If communication is good and the cultures are shared, hints may be adequate. A little silence, a brief stare are often enough to let someone know that he or she has crossed a line.

There are two situations where hints do not work. A predator, even a low-level predator like a passive-aggressive co-worker, may pretend not to see the hints in order to push and make you either vulnerable or at least feel vulnerable. The second situation is dealing with people from different cultures or people who were never socialized into your culture.

In either case, you must set boundaries and they must be stated explicitly. Doing so can be very uncomfortable for most people. Telling people the rules, especially when they should already know them, sounds bossy and places you in a "parent" role. Low-level predators will use this feeling against you: "What's up your ass today? When did you get so insecure?"

Replying with reasons is what the predator wants. As long as you are responding, it is a negotiation and the predator still has some control. Boundary-setting is *never* a negotiation. The only additional information should be a clear statement of the penalty.

"I've told you to leave the door open when you come into my office."

"What's your problem? Are you afraid to be alone with me?" Trying to joke, trying to make the boundary setter defensive. Do you see the predator dynamic here?

"Open the door." Simple, direct statement. No argument, no reasoning, nothing in the voice that could turn it into a question. One of the worst phrases is "I need you to do X for me" as it places all the power on the threat and sounds like a plea on two levels, "need" and "for me." Do not use this tactic when dealing with potential predators. It will backfire.

"Whatever. I wanted to talk to you about..." Disregarding "no" or pretending to ignore boundaries is a huge red flag that you are dealing with a predator.

"Open the door." Staying on message.

"Geeze, can't you stay on the subject?" Again, trying to shift

blame/responsibility, implying that the predator is the one who wants to get the job done and the potential victim is hung up on something minor.

"Open the door or I will file that complaint. Now!" The only thing added to the statement of boundaries is the penalty. "Now" acts as an ultimatum. Once you take this verbal step you must be ready to act on your threat. If the threat ignores you (some will, most won't) and you fail to follow through, you will have marked yourself as easy meat.

We're not going to pretend that a scenario like this will end well every time. Predators are often very successful in an office environment, playing passive-aggressive games and using low-level bullying tactics. The threat will open the door, do his business—and as soon as he leaves tell everyone who will listen, "You won't believe this. That bitch in the office threatened to write me up for closing a door."

Setting boundaries with the very young, the mentally ill, different cultures, or improperly socialized individuals is a little different. (Some kids raised in poverty or foster care or with extremely dysfunctional parents have simply never learned certain social rules, even fundamental stuff like how long to shake hands, or appropriate and inappropriate eye contact.) You still must be very clear and direct. Unlike low-level predators, this group usually appreciates an explanation.

The Iraqi officer said, "If you have a daughter, I would like to marry her."

I took it as a compliment. It was out of the question, of course. A fifteen-year-old bride might be acceptable in the Middle East, but it wouldn't fly at home. Still, my daughter could brag forever that she had her first marriage proposal at fifteen.

"I'll ask her," I said. "See what she thinks. Can I send her your picture?"

"Oh, no, no." He seemed very embarrassed and ended the conversation faster than usual. I looked at D. H., my translator. He shook his head.

"Over here," he explained, "Women don't have anything to do with the negotiation. We don't get that."

"Oh, well in America..."

"He would be okay with you saying 'no'. It would be very bad to have a woman tell him 'no'. Do you see?" I, being socially retarded by Arabic standards, did appreciate the explanation.

Ask, Advise, Order, and Check

This is a cop thing, but it works well whenever you are in a position of authority, including dealing with children. Ask, advise, and order are the standards. The check phrase is an advanced technique that works really well.

- Ask: "*Sir, please lie down on your belly and spread your arms to the side.*" It works most of the time. To change this to kids, just replace the 'sir' with a name and change the instruction to something more relevant such as cleaning up a room or doing the dishes.
- Advise: "*Sir, if you don't lie down on your belly and put your arms out, I will have to use force...*" I usually describe the force I am authorized to use, like a Taser. In some instances that were very high risk, the description might even be, "I'm going to get a group of officers, armor up, and we're going to go in there and pepper spray you, slam you into the ground, and drag you out. I heartily advise you to simply surrender."
- Order: "*Get down! Get down now!*" Strangely enough, I have had more success with the order step than the advise step, even when the advice included some pretty graphic descriptions. At this point, for an officer, force is authorized. However, I've learned to add a check phrase.
- Check: "*So, sir, you're telling me I have no choice but to use force and that is what you choose. Thank you. That makes my paperwork very clear.*" With a kid threatened with a timeout, simply, "Jay you want a time out then? Okay." The beauty of the check phrase is that if you give them just a few seconds to think they realize that they are completely responsible for what is about to happen. Most, in my experience, change their minds and decide to be good.

The ask/advise/order/check protocol is an excellent example of boundary-setting.

Altered States of Mind

We will refer to threats in this subsection as "EDPs." That's cop-speak for Emotionally Disturbed Persons. They can still be threats. The special danger in EDPs is that they are far less predictable than most people. Not always more dangerous or more violent than normal, but harder to see in advance if violence is on the table.

People who are very angry or afraid, mentally ill, or under the influence of drugs do not think like other people. Dealing with altered states of consciousness presents some challenges.

Firstly, this is not something you want to get involved in unless you have no choice. One of the big fears we have when we write a book like this is that someone will decide that reading is enough and walk into a situation that he or she could and should have walked away from. A few hours of reading will never protect you from your own bad decisions.

Secondly, now that that is out of the way, you must also set your goal. Why are you engaging? To talk them down? To talk yourself into a position to escape? To find out what is going on? To try to stabilize them for a few minutes until help can arrive? Once you start talking, you may get emotionally bonded. Double-check yourself to make sure you are still working toward your goal.

Thirdly, it would be very convenient if criminals were criminals and EDPs were EDPs. Someone can be schizophrenic or autistic or have almost any mental disorder you can name and still be a predator. Some people have a tendency to raise their guard when dealing with an EDP, to become a little more scared. Sometimes they also lower their guard in a different area. "Harmless" crazy people can also be thieves or conmen who have a long history of faking mental illness to put victims off guard. Be aware.

Here are some additional concepts to keep in mind:

- A truly mentally ill person does not have a chance to choose his actions. A schizophrenic sees and hears what a schizophrenic sees and hears. There is no choice in the matter and so there is damn little choice in what he can do about it. A person with severe obsessive compulsive order does not want to stop and alphabetize all the books on a shelf or flush every toilet in a public restroom in order; they can fight it for a while, sometimes, but they do not have control.

- One of the signs that someone is faking is control. A truly mentally ill person tries very hard to be normal. They usually don't talk about problems until they trust you. If someone makes a point of telling you, as a stranger, about his mental illness (which is a deeply personal issue), be on your guard.
- Mentally ill does not mean stupid. Do not treat them like children or idiots.
- Do not take what they say personally. Do not get caught in a monkey dance.
- Do not get caught up in the drama of their lives. There are exceptions, such as friends and relatives, but for the most part very few people are prepared for the sacrifices necessary to make a relationship with a severely emotionally disturbed person work.
- Be prepared at all times for sudden changes, including explosive violence.

Much of what has been covered already, including RTPV and listening, are critical in dealing with EDPs. Slow, quiet, and low-pitched (think soothing, but not patronizing) are important. When listening, the goals are twofold: to get a sense of the EDP's internal logic and to find the common ground.

Mental illness and other states that mimic it like drugs and extremely emotional outbreaks are not some hodgepodge where the rules change every second. The person will have an underlying belief about how the world works that includes and explains what they are seeing and feeling. As you get a handle on this internal logic, you will get better at predicting when things will become dangerous.

Do not challenge delusions or dismiss what the EDP is thinking or feeling or seeing. If a schizophrenic is seeing blue men, he or she is seeing blue men. Not pretending, not imagining. The blue men are seen just as clearly as the book you are reading right now. Sometimes with drugs, you can challenge the delusion. If a guy on meth is convinced everyone is trying to kill him, telling him he has taken too much meth might help, but it will work better if he figures that out himself.

So you work from the common ground. "Carl, you know I can't see the blue people, so let's talk about what we both *can* see." Don't patronize. With the exception of the first episodes of adult-onset mental illness or someone who has been drugged, crazy people know that they are crazy. If you pretend to share the delusion, they know you are lying. It destroys trust.

Many people have lived with their mental illnesses or addictions for most of their lives. Respect that. They have survived and often thrive with a problem that might easily have crushed someone else. They can be their own best resource. Co-opt: "Carl, you've dealt with this your whole life. Has it ever been this bad before? What did you do then? What can we do now? How can I help?"

Here are some tactics and tips for dealing with EDPs:

- Match the initial energy. As long as it is not too weird or dangerous, enter the conversation at their level of intensity. If the EDP is pacing, pace alongside. If the EDP is sitting on the floor, humming and rocking, sit next to them, far enough away that they won't see you as a threat. Stay in their peripheral vision. Do not hum and rock, however. Sitting is normal behavior. Pacing is normal behavior. Rocking and humming is not and it will look like you are mocking.
- Once you have started talking, slow down. If you were pacing fast before, slow down and the EDP will usually both slow down to match your pace and calm down to a degree.
- Avoid direct eye contact. Especially with autistics, but for any EDP who is running on fear or anger or drugs (primarily stimulants) that mimic the signs of fear or anger (gross motor activity, elevated blood pressure, etc.), direct eye contact is often interpreted as threat behavior. Practice using your peripheral vision.
- Use positive speech. This is not cheerleader pep talk. Positive speech is simple and directive. Tell them what to do. Avoid telling them what not to do. Say, "Talk quietly," instead of, "Don't be loud."
- Keep things simple. Small words, short sentences. Listening is the most important. If you are listening, the threat is talking. If he is talking, he's not attacking. So far, so good.

- Set clear boundaries. This topic has already discussed in the section titled "Boundaries" above. There is an additional aspect with EDPs, especially the mentally ill. They want to be normal and, if they trust you and like you, they will work their asses off to be normal around you. Friends are rare and they will work to keep friends. This also means that they will be looking to you for advice on what normal is and how to act. Part of learning normal is making implicit boundaries and rules explicit.
- Give them control. Being out of control of your own mind means the world as well is out of your control. Feeling helpless like this is terrible. Whenever you can, show the EDP what he or she *can* control. "I know she made you angry. You can't help that. But you don't have to show her you are angry. Then she will think that she's won." Small steps of self-control have big payoffs, both for the EDP and for you.

Mark was once the subject of a two-page special feature in the local paper about the failure of the mental health care system. Over three hundred pounds and aggressive, Mark was paranoid schizophrenic, bipolar, and learning disabled. He was constantly in and out of custody in our county and the neighboring counties, notorious for staff assaults, and put in Administrative Segregation—where we put the people with a history of extreme violence or other reasons, like intel on a possible escape attempt—and needing to be moved with multiple deputies.

Five or six years ago we'd just started an "open booking" process. Instead of going from cell to cell to cell, constantly either restrained by handcuffs or contained in a cell, we were experimenting with booking fresh arrestees in a setting that looked like an airport waiting area. There were a handful of 'Separation Cells' for special situations, but otherwise there was no secure containment.

We were a little nervous, of course. Open booking (or direct supervision) is the ultimate test of people skills and it usually works well, but the math is bad. Five deputies and one sergeant (all unarmed) responsible for controlling as many as fifty arrestees, most still drunk, high, angry, delusional without any containment or separation.

That night Mark came in. Mark usually left jail into the care of a social worker, and came right back to jail when he threatened or assaulted the social worker.

I talked him through the basic process: search, fingerprinting, digital picture, medical assessment, and interviews with classification and release officers. Within a few minutes of sitting in the common area, he was glaring at a female inmate, mumbling.

I sat down next to him, in the inmate chairs.

"She's looking at me, Sarge. I'm gonna lose it. Make her stop looking at me or I'm going tear her up."

"Mark, you're letting her get to you. Yes she's staring at you, but if you react, you'll be the one to get in trouble. Don't let her control you."

"She's laughing at me!"

"And if you go off, she wins, Mark. Don't let her win. Ignore her. Show her she can't get to you."

The other inmate was laughing at Mark. Mark was huge, greasy, filthy. Like a lot of schizophrenics and developmentally disabled, he couldn't take care of himself. I took the other inmate aside and told her that Mark was "retarded" and it wasn't his fault and it was cruel to laugh at him. She apologized.

I spent probably an hour with Mark, kept him calm. Then I went to lunch. Within five minutes, the call came over the radio, "Sarge, one to sep." Mark was going to a Separation Cell.

When I arrived, he was screaming and kicking the steel door, frothing at the mouth and yelling death threats. I keyed the door open, stepped in and asked him to have a seat. I listened, mostly, but I stayed on message. "You need to calm down. I have civilians like the nurse out there and I will not let you out of this cell if you are acting out in any way."

It dawned on Mark that he outweighed me by over a hundred pounds and I was alone with him in a tiny concrete cell and showing no fear. You could see him try to puzzle it out, using all of his available cunning to guess what my secret security came from…

He asked a lot of questions and finally asked if I'd been in the military. I said, "Yeah. Army." And he relaxed. This poor kid, who never got any closer to the service than a Rambo movie, relaxed. I wasn't afraid because I was a soldier. Of course.

I remember him trying to remember everything he was taught in therapy and classes about socializing, about how normal people make friends and Mark reached out to ask a question, the kind of question he imagined friends asked friends, "So what did you like best about the Army? Living in the barracks with all the guys or the uniforms?"

"Honestly, Mark, the only thing I miss was crawling around in the mud and shooting people. I enjoyed that." On one level, that was a screwed up thing to say, truth or not. But it gave me one of the best moments in my career.

Mark said, "Man, that's not right. You should talk to someone about that." Mark, the paranoid/schizophrenic, bipolar, developmentally disabled, violent and assaultive criminal was giving me fatherly advice. He recommended a counselor.

We talked some more, and he promised to be quiet and keep control even when I wasn't there watching. He kept his word all the way up to housing.

**

I found out a couple years ago that Mark had died. I don't know when or where or the exact circumstances; it was just one of those passing comments in briefing: "By the way, they found Mark R. dead a couple of weeks ago."

He probably died alone. Hypothermia or OD on an attempt to "self-medicate" or maybe his diabetes got out of control. I wonder who knows or cares; who, outside of a handful of social workers and jail guards remember him. I wonder if anyone else has a good memory of Mark.

Cold Conversation Drill

Talking is talking, and if you are like most people, you probably do too much. There is an exercise we want to leave you with. For the next week or month or year, possibly for the rest of your life if you get addicted, we want you to strike up a conversation with a stranger.

To get you started, observe the stranger and look for a hook, something specific and preferably personal: "That looks like a good book." "Where was the picture on your desk taken?" "I noticed your shoes. Are you a runner?" Then shut up and listen. People love to talk about themselves and many are fascinating—but you have to listen.

The cold conversation is a skill and it will improve with time. You will learn how to ask questions and how to give enough information yourself to keep things flowing.

> "Oana, I can't place your accent. Where are you from?"
>
> She grinned evilly and made claws with her fingers. Emphasizing the accent she said, "I am from Transylvania."
>
> "Really? I heard the Carpathian Mountains are beautiful."
>
> "You know of the Carpathians? Let me tell you..."

Voice is the second lowest level of the six force options, but it is arguably the most important. Unless you work in certain high-risk professions or are really unlucky, the chances of your needing to face violence on any given day are pretty small. But everyone communicates with others all the time. There's no down side to being good at it.

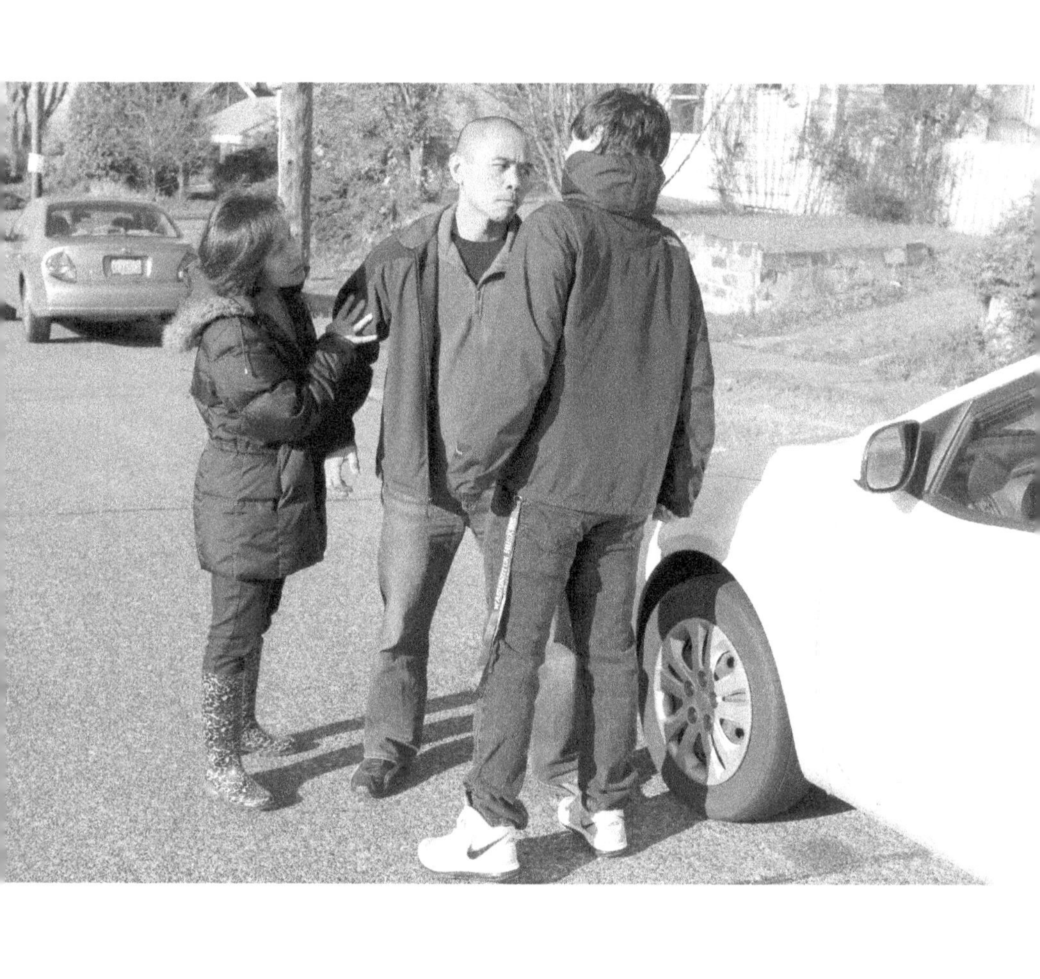

LEVEL 3—TOUCH

Touch is a quasi-level. It is still communication, still attempting to influence instead of force, but it involves laying hands on someone without permission. That makes it legally fuzzy, since "good" touch and "bad" touch can very much be a matter of interpretation. We all know the power of a touch, a hug that calms a frightened child, or a quick grip on the shoulder in a moment of grief or indecision. It can be a communication beyond words.

Touching can also be a mistake.

Touching, at any level, is also something that an experienced threat can use as a hook:

> The two brothers had backed me up against a fence. It was late, I was on my way home from work, and I was triangulated. One reached for my chest and I gently parried the hand away, trying to be smiling and conversational: "Just on my way home guys, don't have time..."
>
> When I parried his reaching hand away he snarled, "Don't touch me!" and swung. The fight was on.

Unless you know the subject well, touch has the possibility to trigger memories that you cannot be aware of. It is generally ineffective to comfort a stranger who has been raped by enfolding her in a big hug. In most cultures world-wide, touching across genders is never appropriate between strangers. Outside of the US and Northern Europe, even shaking hands, wait for the woman to offer her hand first. The same thing goes for certain orthodox religious communities in the US today.

You must be aware that touching has taboos. Unless you are attempting to dominate someone on a massive scale, you do not touch him or her above the shoulders. Placing a hand on the head or the neck is something done to children or lovers at times; otherwise it will have a very bad reaction. It shows dominance or intimacy.

Touching may also be a bad strategic decision. You cannot touch without being in the threat's striking range. Because of the action/reaction gap (your ability to defend will rarely be fast enough for an non-telegraphed, close-range attack), you are extremely vulnerable. Attempting to handle a potentially hostile or volatile threat with touch is betting everything on your skill at reading intent. If you are wrong, expect to bleed.

In a potentially volatile situation, any touch must be done with respect for your own safety. To look into someone's eyes while placing a manly hand on the shoulder puts almost all of your best targets right in range, takes one of your arms out of the defensive mix, and may trigger explosive action. It is not a safe move.

As long as you don't surprise the threat, it is actually less likely to trigger an emotional response if you approach from the side. Remember in "Presence," discussing proxemics? The intimate/threat ranges are measured face-to-face. People can stand far more comfortably with strangers behind or to the sides. That may not make strategic sense, but look at the way people stand in crowded elevators.

The ideal contact point for a touch is the back of the elbow. The distal end of the humerus is the maximum leverage you can put on the arm and, although there are limits, with that one contact point you can either move a much bigger and stronger person or prevent that person from moving. The natural motion against the leverage point, pushing the threat's arm across his body, also rotates him around his spine and puts you on his rear flank, one of the best places to be in a fight, should a fight happen.

If you go to touch, be prepared at all times for things to go bad.

Generally, there are effectively four ways to use touch: calming, directive, distractive, and projection.

Calming Touch

Calming touch ranges from patting someone's hand (something you see at funerals a lot) all the way up to a hug. It is just making a human connection with another human who you feel is dealing with pain, fear, grief, or anger. It must be sincere. The reason that the manly hand on the shoulder and direct eye contact leaves you so vulnerable is because there is no way to blade the body and place your off hand in a defensive position that does not ruin the comforting effect.

Calming is about sharing and thus diffusing emotion, making people feel safe enough that they do not have to do anything immediately and thus giving time for the adrenaline (or drugs) to leave the system. **You cannot calm someone down if you look like you are preparing for combat.** Any calming touch must be done with a caring demeanor and usually backed with sincere and sympathetic words presented in a low, slow, quiet voice.

Calming touch will succeed or fail depending on your read of the situation, your timing, and your social skills. Calming touch only has a chance to be effective when you are dealing with emotion. You cannot hug a mugger and make him feel so much better about himself that he won't mug you. If he is mugging you for money to buy drugs to stave off withdrawals, a hug really does not fill that gap.

So first, read the situation. Number one, is this an emotional threat? Number two, is it the kind of emotional threat that can be calmed by touch? The Monkey Dance is emotional, but it is damnably hard to hug your way out of.

Is this really your problem? Notice that we ask that a lot? Are you the one to deal with it at all and, if so, do you have the relationship or is this the type of situation where calming touch will work?

The reason touch is a quasi-level is because there are so few situations where it is appropriate, so few where it might work, and the majority of those are things you could walk away from with no ill effects.

There are two exceptions:

Rory has comforted suicidal people. That may sound cool, but it is dangerous as all hell. Suicide is homicide and if someone really wants to kill himself, he has already gotten over the social conditioning and moral issues of killing a person. That includes you. Touch may help here, to build rapport, and put you in a position to disarm or disable the threat, but do not for a second think that because someone wants to kill himself, he would hesitate to kill you.

The other exception is that touch can be used for absolute naked intimidation. What we said before about not hugging your way out of a monkey dance? Once upon a time, there was a guy going off, swinging his arms, calling the officer's "cocksuckers," and daring them to fight. Rory walked over, gave him a hug and told him he "may want to rephrase that." That is possibly the most he has ever scared a human being. The arrestee was extremely polite for the rest of his time in custody.

Directive Touch

Directive touch is simply steering. A light hand on the back or the elbow-leverage-control point and you direct the stumbling drunk toward the exit. Of the touch level variations, directive touch is the most likely to be effective and safe.

You are close, so you must be prepared for things to go bad, but most steering positions put you in a safer situation than trying to comfort. Applying directive touch, especially with a drunk, is the crisis point. If the drunk was planning on leaving quietly, he would have left when presented with presence (the bouncers show up) or verbal, "Sir, you need to leave." That he did not presents the possibility that resisting might be on his mind. When directive touch is applied, you will know for sure, one way or the other.

There is no leverage applied or pain compliance with directive. If that needs to happen, you have jumped to Level 4. This is just simple guidance.

Distractive Touch

If you've ever had your significant other kick you under the table to keep you from saying something stupid, you are already familiar with distractive touch. People pay attention to touches, even when they should be paying attention to something else. Sometimes it makes them shut up, usually it makes them look to see who is touching them and why.

Distractive touch is used to bring the threat's attention to you or a part of you. If the threat is focused on someone he intends to hurt and you tap on his shoulder, the threat will turn to you. His intended victim can escape. The obvious downside of this is that once his intention turns to you, you might become the new intended victim. You must read the situation to determine if this is likely and whether you can handle it.

Distraction, unlike calming, can be used as a surprise and often works better that way. Watching a cat stalking, you see a perfect predator: graceful, efficient, all senses well beyond what a human can do, and totally focused. It is easy as anything to sneak up on a cat that is stalking something else and grab its tail, and the cat will jump in complete surprise. People are similar, and often any serious surprise can disrupt the most hardened predator.

But USE YOUR HEAD! While it is true that an unexpected touch can disrupt a human threat or a cat, so can a shout, and a shout can be done at a safer distance. Sneaking up on cats is cool. It applies to people. Nowhere in that set of facts is any indicator that it is the best way.

Distraction can also be used to make lower levels of force work. Many martial arts teach a light, distracting blow before applying a lock. You must be careful, because the law does not really distinguish between a "distracting blow to the head" and any other "blow to the head." Using a Level 5 technique to make a Level 4 technique work is decent, tactically, but legally you have to justify the Level 5—and if you can justify Level 5, you need Level 5. What the hell are you doing at Level 4?

Projecting Touch

It was my last week working the jail before leaving for Iraq. I kind of wanted something epic to happen, just to say goodbye. So I was eager for the backup call and took off at a sprint. By the time I got there, the incident was controlled. The threat, a very big, experienced con, had let himself be handcuffed. I walked him to the disciplinary cells.

One of the downsides of working with a really professional force is that sometimes the inmates aren't used to it. They expect to get their asses kicked and when we don't, they sometimes mistakenly assume it is weakness. As I walked the inmate to his new cell, he got more aggressive, trying to push and pull and talk some pretty wild shit. In the enclosed cell, I had him put his head against the wall to disrupt his balance and started to take the cuffs off.

As soon as the first one came off, he surged off the wall twisting and swinging. I just pressed in and up under and behind his armpit before he could complete the spin. He found himself helpless, barely balanced on one foot. Not only could he not turn or punch, but he couldn't even put his foot down. His balance was so shot that a slight push would plant his head in the concrete wall, and an out, up and downward tug would face plant him in the floor.

I kept my voice calm, deadpan, as if he hadn't just attempted an assault, "Sir, it's usually a bad idea to move fast, especially when the cuffs come off. Just one officer in here, I might misinterpret and over-react. Okay?"

"Good advice, sarge."

Projection gets into a very fuzzy area. There are ways to apply a very light force or simply to direct the force the threat is applying that can have serious effects but do not fit neatly into control or pain or damage categories. If someone punches you in the face and you barely tap it so that he misses your head and shatters his fist against the wall, what level of force have you used? Less energy was expended than in simply steering a drunk. Making him miss your face protected both you and the fragile bones of his hand (if there is no wall or similarly solid object behind you) and had intent similar to keeping a drunk from stumbling into a wall.

The cool thing about projections, though, is that they are a very low level of force that can work particularly well for one of the primary goals in self-defense: getting away. **Perfect projection is nothing more than getting out of the way skillfully.**

In this sense, projections are ways to move a threat or get the other guy to move with minimum force and without applying that force to any part of the threat's body likely to result in injury.

There are three principles to making projections work:

- Use the threat's momentum.
- Use the threat's structure.
- Control the threat's contact with the ground.

Whenever the threat moves, whether pushing, pulling, or charging, he is putting energy into the world. That energy has a strength and a direction. To stop the strength requires at least as much energy. Changing the direction, however, requires very little power. The more strength, in many ways, the easier it is to misdirect the power.

As an example, imagine a baseball bat swung at your head. In order to stop the force with your forearm, you would have to hit the bat at least as hard as the bat is hitting you. Further, your arm would have to be sturdy enough to withstand the combined force of the bat and your block, not just one of those forces, both. On the good side, when your forearm shatters, the bone breaking will bleed off some of the energy of the bat. Your floppy shattered arm sticking to the bat will add some drag, slowing the bat even more and when the combination of forces from your shattered arm and misshapen broken skull equal the power of the baseball bat swing, the bat will come to a stop. Congratulations.

The same swing, tapped at a ninety-degree angle to the direction of travel will jump off of its intended plane. In other words, it will miss with a relatively small application of force. That's kindergarten stuff.

Power applied to the side and with a drawing motion, keeping the bat as close to the intended plane as possible while still missing and adding to the momentum, transfers the force both from the swing and your draw or pull to the threat. The threat loses his balance.

That is just an illustration, but this is one of the primary principles of projecting: The threat does the work. Not you.

Second, use structure. Structure is a way to maximize leverage and use bones to move other bones. If you push on the side of a big man's stomach, the flesh will squish out of the way. If you push on his shoulder or hip with the same power, his body will twist.

Shoulder girdle and pelvis are both fairly rigid and attached to each other through the spine. They act as lever arms to control the spine and as such can manipulate each other as well as arms and legs. Sound complicated? If someone goes to kick with his right foot and you press down on his right shoulder, he has to abort the kick and put his foot on the ground to avoid falling. Now add that 'drawing' aspect mentioned above and you can really toy with someone.

In the example at the start of this section, when the inmate turned on Rory, Rory knew he could not beat the guy's strength. He was just too big. But a light push up and under the armpit used the shoulder girdle as a lever arm to force the spine sideways. A sideways tilt to the spine forces one foot to dangle in the air and, with the spine extended, robs the threat of any core strength. Even if he were a good kicker, in that position he couldn't develop power.

Using your own structure—a continuous chain of power from the ground to your point of contact—is too big a subject to go into here. If you're interested in delving deeply into the power chain, how to align the body to hit with maximum force, consider *The Way of Sanchin Kata* (both book and DVD) by Kris Wilder. Suffice to say that whenever possible, you want to hit with bone and if someone tries to push you, you want them pushing rigid bone instead of muscle. Unless, of course, you want to just evade the force and project the threat into a wall.

The last principle is to control the threat's contact with the ground. Our first impulse was to say "disrupt the threat's contact with the ground" and that is true most of the time. However, in the example that opens this section, one of the threat's feet was actually trapped on the ground.

Most projections will have a sideways vector (to make the incoming attack miss) and a drawing vector (that disguises the fact of a miss, adds force to the miss, and subtly disrupts the person's instinctive way to control the force). If you add even a slight upward vector, the drawing force (especially if the threat is putting a lot of power in) can take the threat completely off his feet.

So how are projections used in self-defense? Most of the time they are used for escaping. When an attack comes in and you shift to the side or the threat focuses away, or you choose to intervene in an attack on a third party, sometimes a simple push in the right direction will give you space and time to escape, something that might be far more difficult to accomplish using fists and elbows.

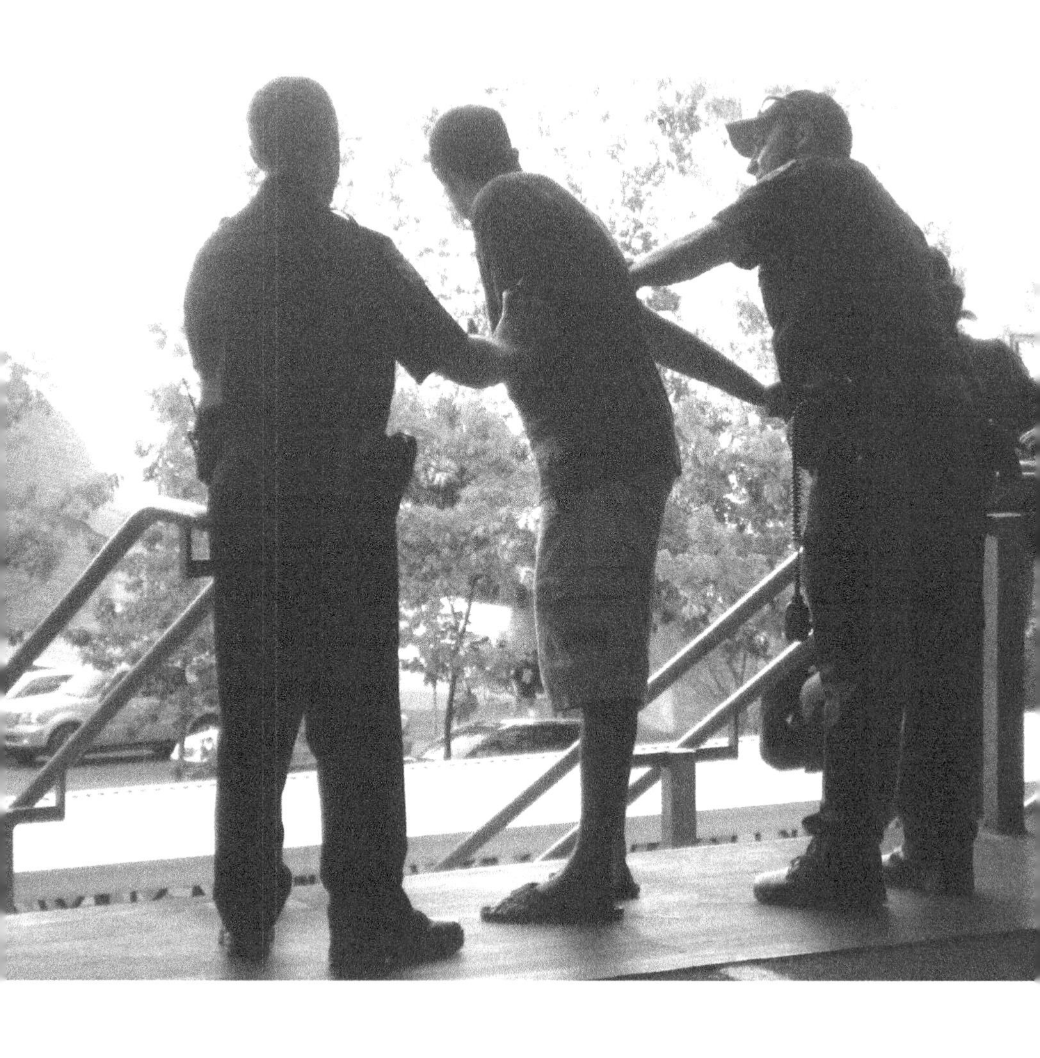

INTERLUDE—ARE YOU READY FOR LEVEL 4?

Levels one through three are essentially communication. At Level 3, touch, even though you are placing hands on the threat, you are demonstrably guiding, assisting, or comforting. At Level 4, you are placing hands on the other guy, but what you are doing, if not legally justified, is assault. You are going to *force* the adversary to move or to stop moving or, through pain, *influence* the other guy to move or stop moving.

This, ladies and gentlemen, is a crime. You may only do this if your justifications are clear. Not just clear to you in your emotional state at the time, but something you can make clear, if necessary, to a jury.

Level 4, while ubiquitous in the tournament ring, should be the rarest of self-defense skills. The locks, takedowns, holds, and pressure points common at this level are rarely fight-enders. They do not stop the threat so much as *discourage* the threat. Unless you break the joint (a higher level of force), a joint lock merely discourages a threat. You cannot hold the lock forever, and when you let go, the other guy is completely capable of attacking again.

As such, though locks and pins temporarily take away means, they depend on altering intent. That works best on weak intent.

Level 4 techniques are also unlikely to work against an aggressive, dangerous threat. It is very hard to actually snatch an incoming fist out of the air and apply a lock. It is difficult and dangerous to close on a knife for a takedown. Pressure points do not work nearly as well on infuriated threats as they do on eager, curious classmates.

These factors combine to make Level 4 rare outside of the law enforcement and security communities. Specifically, Level 4 techniques are not fight-enders, work best against less-dedicated threats, and are difficult to pull off without getting hurt. Civilians do not have a duty to act, so most things that can be handled at Level 4 can also be handled by walking away.

That bears repeating: **Most things that can be handled at Level 4 can also be handled by walking away.**

Most often, in a civilian setting, Level 4 will be used on people you don't want to hurt, your friends and relatives. These are people who are unlikely to sue you or press charges anyway. Breaking up a fight at a family picnic, taking the keys from your inebriated roommate, immobilizing an out-of-control child, these are all legitimate uses of Level 4. Attempting to disarm a drug-crazed lunatic is not.

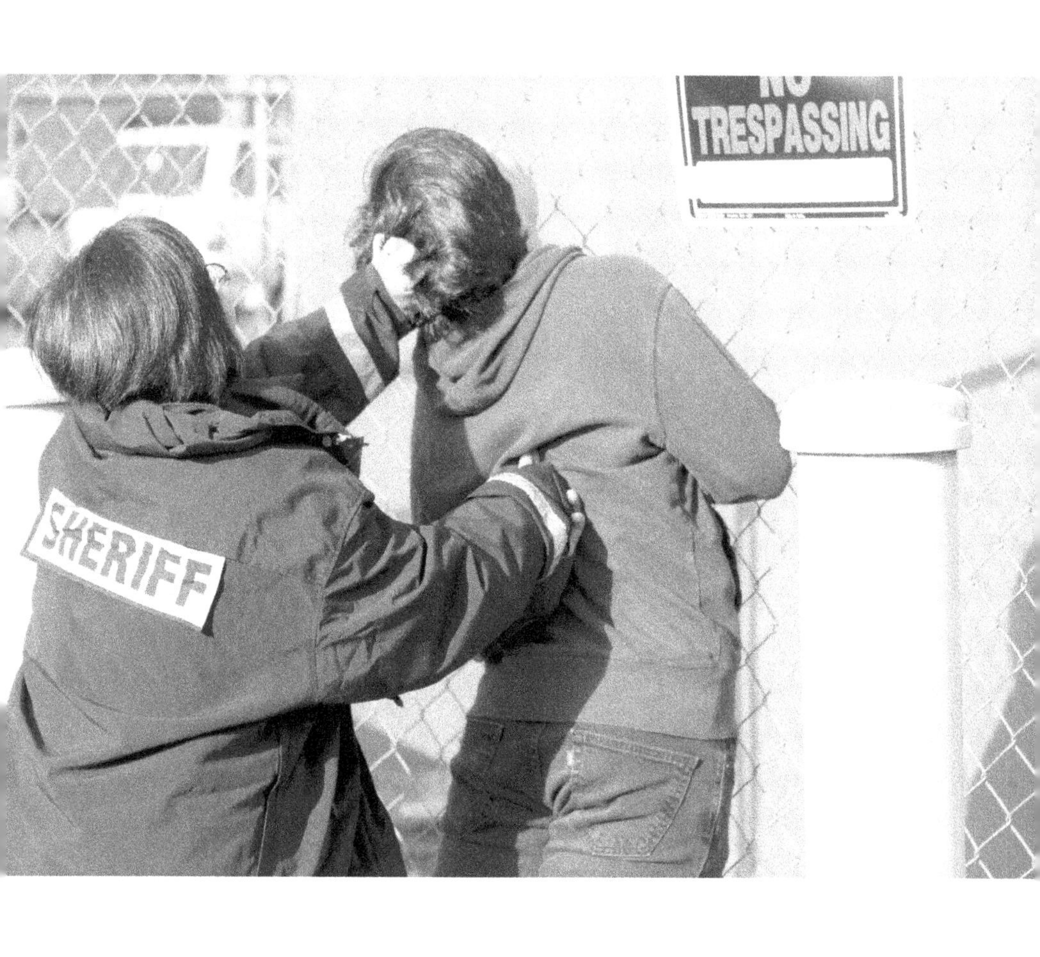
TRESPASSING
SHERIFF

LEVEL 4—EMPTY-HAND RESTRAINT/PHYSICAL CONTROL

Level 4 includes a wide variety of techniques that are designed to gain compliance through pain or force compliance through leverage, with a relatively low risk of injury. Even though you are not intending to do lasting harm to the other guy, if you use these techniques in the wrong circumstances, you are very likely to be charged with a crime (e.g., assault, unlawful imprisonment).

The techniques will only stop a fight temporarily at best. Pain points hurt, but that's all. If the pain does not wilt the attacker, the fight is still on, possibly with more rage thrown into the mix. Joint locks hurt and can either force or prevent movement, but you must either let them go, break the joint, or wait for help to arrive. That may take some time, perhaps a *lot* of time. If you have someone under control, a break or dislocation requires a whole new level of justification.

Under what circumstances could you show that someone in a lock was still an immediate threat to the degree that serious injury was appropriate? Not a rhetorical question. When we throw these questions out, think them through. In this instance, if you have someone locked up and they draw a knife with the other hand, you betcha a broken joint becomes justified.

As such, Level 4 is appropriate when you are very, very confident that you will prevail. If it turns out to be false confidence and things go sideways, they will go sideways very quickly. By attempting to apply a Level 4 technique, just like at Level 3, you are very close, well within reach of the threat. The very fact that you were sure you could handle it at this level indicates that you will be surprised when you fail.

If you decide to go in at Level 4, **be prepared to immediately jump to a higher level if you start taking damage.** Do not hesitate.

Joint Locks

What I love about teaching cops is that they have absolutely no bullshit threshold. If something works, fine. If not, don't waste their time. I was advocating small joint locks for our deputies, specifically expanding our DTs to work fingerlocks. When it was demo time, Ski stepped up. About six foot ten, over three-hundred pounds, he used to play the line for a professional football team. Shit.

I shook my head sadly and went to shake his hand. He responded and I turned my hand, catching one of his massive fingers in the web of my thumb and wrapping my little and ring fingers over the joint in his index finger. I immediately pulled forward and down, careful to keep pressure on.

In a second, Ski was stretched out on the floor, arm fully extended. I was stretched out as well, facing him. Staring into his cold blue eyes.

"It's a good thing I love you like a brother," he said, "because if I didn't I'd kick your ass as soon as you let go."

People overcomplicate joint locks. We're aware of one style that claims to have over three hundred named wristlocks. Impressive. Looked at from another point of view, since there are only eight possible ways to lock the wrist, it seems pretty excessive.

Here's the skinny on locks. There are only three kinds of joints in the human body that can be locked:

- Ball and socket (shoulder, hip, base of the fingers and toes)
- Hinge (elbow, knee, and finger)
- Gliding (wrist)

We are staying away from the spine, because a spine lock is a Level 6 (lethal force) technique. We also did not mention the ankle. It's a gliding joint, like the wrist, but so muscle-bound that torque applied to the ankle almost always threatens the knee instead.

Each type of joint locks in the same way. A hinge joint lock works by hyperextension. A ball-and-socket lock works by rotation on a lever arm. A gliding joint works by applying force, preferably along two planes simultaneously. Simple, right? It is. Don't get caught in the big words and concepts. Understanding locks is a much faster way to apply them in a fight than memorizing locks.

There are a few principles that make all locks work. The two most important for applying locks in a dynamic situation (like a fight) are gifts and basing.

Gifts

The only way you will get a lock or a takedown is if the other guy gives it to you. Take heart. The beauty of these classes of techniques is that the threat is always giving you *something*; you just have to learn to see it.

For an example, unless you are much, much stronger than the other guy, you will never get an elbowlock on an adversary who is pulling his arms in. If he pushes, however, he is giving you the elbowlock. You just have to apply it. The pulling that negates the elbowlock sets up the shoulderlock and often the wristlock. The key skill to applying locks (and takedowns) in real life is the ability to recognize and exploit the gifts that the threat presents.

Basing

A lock is only a lock if the threat is moving or is based. You cannot hold a lock in the air unless the threat lets you. In every simple lock, there is a natural direction to move that makes the lock disappear. To combat this, you must be able to move the lock fast enough to keep the force ahead of the threat or plant the threat into a hard surface, such as the floor or a wall, so that he does not have weasel room to escape from the lock.

Putting the threat into a hard surface is called basing. A variant of basing is stacking, where you apply two locks that work in different directions. An example is a shoulderlock with finger assist.

Leverage

Maximizing your leverage is basic physics. The longer the lever arm, the more force you can apply. When applying a lock to the elbow, you want one hand on or just above the joint (the fulcrum of the lever) and the other as far down the arm as you can get, until you hit the wrist. As your hand moves toward the wrist, the lever arm becomes longer and the technique more effective. As it moves closer to the elbow, the lever arm becomes shorter and the technique less effective. With a twisting wristlock, your longest lever arm is diagonally across the back of the hand.

Let gravity do your work for you whenever possible. Try to keep your body weight over your technique. In an emergency, you can even drop your full weight onto a lock.

Two-way action

Two-way action is one of the fundamentals of Wally Jay's *Small Circle Jujitsu*. It is critical. Many people are taught to immobilize one half of the lock (say the fulcrum) and push or pull with the other. Push *and* pull both ends of the lever. Push the fulcrum *and* pull on the lever arm (or vice versa). It is more than twice as effective as doing either alone.

Applying joint locks

Once you understand the joints, *gifts, basing, leverage*, and *two-way action* are the basics of making a lock work. The next question becomes, how do you use them? Joint locks are versatile and have several purposes.

They hurt, when properly applied. Pain as a specific tool will be addressed under pressure points in the "Specific Points" section below. It is enough for now to say that joint locks cause enough pain that many threats may decide it is not worth the risk to continue to be threats.

When joint locks work, it sends a message. Very, very few people can actually apply a joint lock in a real fight. When you do (and good joint locks, even when accidental, often look effortless), it sometimes gets interpreted that you must be a really, really good fighter. That can make the other guy rethink his decision to start trouble.

Mechanically, locks that are not based are used to make a threat move. Fingerlocks are great for forcing people to stand up. Come-along locks are called "come-alongs" because they make it easy to walk someone out of an establishment. A lock that extends the threat's center of gravity outside of his feet becomes a takedown. Based locks are used to prevent someone from moving, to freeze the threat in place while maintaining your safety until help can arrive.

Lastly, joints are easier to break than bones. To deliberately dislocate a joint is a higher level of force than Level 4. If damage is justified and you have no other options, joint locks can be adapted to higher levels of force. It takes skill, though. Until you learn to see and exploit gifts, it is very, very unlikely that you will be able to pull off a good lock in a full-scale, chaotic brawl.

Hinge joints

Hinge joints include the elbow, knee, and the joints in the middle of the fingers (and toes, but c'mon. How often do you get attacked by a barefoot guy outside the *dojo*? And those little suckers are tough to get a grip on. And they stink). When you see the gift of the extending or extended limb, you apply pressure at two places—the fulcrum point and as far down the lever arm as you can. It is that simple. We can show you dozens and dozens of elbow and knee locks, but they all boil down to that: Apply pressure at two points. Simple.

A food port is the rectangular slot in a steel door in a jail cell that allows particularly dangerous inmates to be fed while keeping others out of arm's reach. Occasionally, inmates try to attack officers, other inmates and, for some reason, especially nurses, by grabbing them through the food port and pulling their arms in to mangle.

Because the inmates in these cells are high-risk, it was policy to cuff them through the food port. It prevented force and injury if the inmate put his hands through and was cuffed before the door was even open.

A particularly dangerous one let one hand get cuffed and then tried to pull my partner's arm through the food port. T. yanked back. I grabbed the threat's arm. I could feel him surging; he had a foot braced against a door. I shifted direction and pressed, putting the back of his elbow against the edge of the food port. The threat continued to fight until his arm was ready to break and then gave up.

Force needs to be applied at two points. That's all. It does not need to be hands or legs. You can apply one or both of the force pressures with your head, shoulder, furniture, or the wall. Even with the threat's own body.

The exception: There is one other way to lock a hinge joint. Because of the way they are constructed, you can place an object in the fulcrum, at the fold (e.g., inner elbow, back of the knee) and bend the joint over it until it pops. The figure-4 leg lock is the best example of this. People often give up because of the pain trying it on an elbow, even when the joint is nowhere close to danger. The fact that fingers have two hinge joints with a length of bone in between allows for a variation of this concept.

Ball-and-Socket Joints

Ball-and-socket joints are almost too easy to write about. But they are hard to apply in action because you have to be very close (which sometimes makes the threat escalate to a higher use of force), and these locks require big motions that frequently tie up both of your hands. So there are disadvantages. That said, they are sometimes effective.

Distal (that means away from the body) to every ball-and-socket joint is a hinge joint. To make a really effective ball-and-socket joint, you bend (or find already bent) the hinge joint to ninety degrees and turn it like a water faucet. The closer the bend is to 90 degrees, the better your leverage. Twisting in one direction will lock the joint faster than the other direction, but both will get a lock.

Remember that only the hand on the leverage point applies force to the lock. The other hand stabilizes the stem of the "water faucet" to maintain the ninety degrees.

There is also an exception to the rule that ball-and-socket joints work from twisting a bent hinge joint. Because of the structure of the hinge joint, you can also create an elevated shoulderlock, using the whole, straight arm to lever the shoulder joint apart. The leverage point on the back of the elbow can also be applied to attack the shoulder in a different direction.

The leverage point on the back of the elbow, the distal end of the humerus, can also be used to lock or tear the shoulder. If the threat's hand is raised (the gift), the leverage point can be pushed up and back. There is a similar dynamic and the same physics in aikido's *shiho nage* (four-direction throw), where the wrist or forearm is pulled down and back to attack the shoulder or take the threat to the ground.

Hips are also ball-and-socket joints. Although the principles are the same, the hip is so strong that in a healthy person, locking the hip will almost always result in just rolling the threat over, not in a great deal of pain or a dislocation.

Gliding Joints

One of the processes when you get arrested if you won't be immediately released is "dress-in." It's different in different facilities, but in this particular case a group of four inmates and two officers went to a separate room. The arrestees stripped off their street clothes, hung them in labeled bags and put on their jail uniforms. Three of them did anyway.

One of them, still drunk, started talking shit, trying to provoke a reaction. You know, "Dickhead" this and "Your mother" that. The usual stuff. Just testing the water.

It was late, we were tired and frankly, we didn't really care. As long as he got in his little jail uniform and we could take him upstairs, and let him sleep it off, he could say anything he wanted.

He didn't see it that way. What he saw was that he wasn't getting his ass kicked, so he started yelling his insults. We were professionals. We were actually bored. This was nothing new. So he still didn't get his ass kicked.

So he took a swing.

I generally don't advocate wristlocks against punches. It takes an incredible edge in speed and precision. But this dude was a little drunk, a lot of stupid, and not particularly fast. It was the very predictable overhand right-looping punch. My hand went cross body in a circle, taking his hand from the outside, parrying it away from me. When he drew his fist back, my hand just stayed where it was, gripped and twisted.

I learned the technique as *sankaju*, but have heard it called *sankyo*. It is a rotational wristlock with the hand down and the elbow above the shoulder, the forearm straight down.

I held it one handed as the inmate tried to jump up and down, yelling and thrashing. I turned to my partner, "You got the rest of these guys, Nick?"

"Yeah. No problem."

I marched him out with the wristlock. He was naked and struggling for all he was worth. I had to march him past a group of other inmates on the way to the separation cell. They started laughing. I made a point of taking a sip of coffee as we walked. That was when he realized that I'd never put down my coffee cup (I didn't have time anyway). He calmed down when he saw that.

The wrist is a gliding joint. There is no bone-in-bone socketing. Applying a wristlock is simply a matter of tightening the ligaments that hold the wrist together. The ligaments can be tightened by bending the wrist or by twisting the wrist. That's it. Bend up, bend down. Twist clockwise, twist counterclockwise. It is almost always more efficient to bend and twist in combination.

Simple, huh? Bend up. Bend down. Twist clockwise. Twist counterclockwise. Bend up and twist clockwise. Bend up and twist counterclockwise. Bend down and twist clockwise. Bend down and twist counterclockwise. There are only eight possible wristlocks, unless you want to get complicated just for the hell of it and bend at different angles.

The hard part about wristlocks is that your gripping surface is usually a fist or a hand that tends to be small, sweaty, and slippery. Hard to grip and hard to apply much leverage to. This challenge makes it critical that you work the gift instead of trying to muscle the lock. If you do muscle the lock, the usual effect is not that the threat gets injured, but that your hands slip off.

If the grip is applied directly to the wrist, your own fingers create a splint and make the wrist stronger and your lock weaker.

Small joints, such as wrists and fingers, are exceptionally effective as pain-compliance techniques. They hurt a lot, which tends to make it easier to use to force a threat to move. Wrists are also rarely injured. No bone is directly affected, so the injury that would be most likely is a pull or tear of the tendons or ligaments. Most people do not have the grip strength to pull this off—their hands will slip before the threat's tendons snap.

From a liability standpoint, that makes wristlocks a great choice and something taught to most officers and many martial artists. The downside is that they are very difficult to pull off against someone who's attacking.

Wristlocks do not have the mechanical leverage or anatomical ability to control the entire body, such as some elbowlocks can do. As such, **if the threat does not respond to pain, you cannot rely on a wristlock.**

If you are unfamiliar with locking, get a partner and play with each other's wrists. See how far you have to twist it before pain occurs. Notice that you may have to twist much farther clockwise than counterclockwise (or vice versa) depending on position. Do the same thing with bending in all directions. Then combine bending with twisting again, all bends plus each possible twist. Practice this from different positions and with different grips. You must rely on your partner for honest feedback.

Repeat the above, but feel where the joint "sticks," where the tendons have tightened to their limits of motion without stretching. This should be very near the point of pain, but it is this feeling you will be looking for when you apply the technique on a threat.

Wristlocks will never be a primary assault survival technique, but they are useful, especially if you can gain surprise, as come-alongs.

Fingerlocks

Fingers are tiny marvels of engineering. And they give many opportunities for play and pain. Each finger is a ball-and-socket joint with two hinge joints and set close enough to other fingers that they can be twisted across each other. In addition, a hard object placed between a threat's fingers and squeezed can give some excruciating pain, and so can any ring a threat happens to be wearing.

Fingers are delicate, easy to break. They are very sensitive to pain in most people, and when a drunk is feeling pain nowhere else, he can often still feel some in his fingers.

Conversely, some fingerlocks are fine motor skills and you may have some difficulty pulling them off under stress. Not always, though. Just latching onto something is a primate stress ability and if it is a finger or two, that's fine. You may not be able to make the threat dance with exquisitely nuanced pressure, but you can still twist the damn things. You may also find in some close fighting, particularly on the ground, that, if the gift presents itself, fingers are easy to latch onto.

To use the hinge joint aspects of the fingers, catch the tip of one or two fingers in the web of your thumb and curl the other fingers over the back of the threat's fingers. The ring finger often makes contact at the point of maximum leverage. If the threat has really large hands, it may be the little finger. Either way, try to keep your other fingers out of the way. If they grip, they act as splints and decrease the effectiveness of the lock.

Maintain constant pressure on both points of contact. Hands are squirrelly and the threat will try to move unless you base him (by planting him in a wall or over a table, for instance) or base the lock, which you can do by pressing the palm of the locked hand against an unmoving surface, including you or the threat. If you cannot base, the easiest way to maintain pressure is to concentrate on pointing your index finger at the threat's elbow.

The reverse of this grip is to get the pads of the threat's fingers into your palm, or under your thumb, and use your other fingers to apply pressure to the joint.

The ball-and-socket joint aspects of fingers can be manipulated by twisting a bent finger. Straight fingers can also be twisted around each other for a similar effect. Fingers are a pretty effective tool. Done right, they can be leveraged to control bigger and more powerful adversaries.

Practicing Joint Locks

The key to using locks in a real situation is to recognize the opportunity to apply the lock. Physical skills are much easier than observational skills.

The Joint Lock Flow Drill requires a partner. It is a non-resisting drill. Both partners stand facing each other. You apply a lock of any kind to your partner (not fast, not hard, don't hurt each other). The partner analyzes the lock and escapes (you do not prevent the escape by changing or adapting; that is not the drill. You must cooperate to learn the most from each other).

The most common ways to escape include going with the pain, sliding the locked limb off one or both of the contact points, or turning/rotating the locked limb at ninety degrees to the lines of pressure. You can use a free limb to apply this technique, but usually the trapped limb can extricate itself.

Once the partner has escaped, both of you will be in a different position. The partner then decides what locks your position presents and goes for the most efficient option. You then escape and the drill repeats for as long as you want. Stay in contact and move slowly enough that you are using technique rather than brute force. Done properly, this becomes a moving drill that will have you locking and escaping locks from a wide variety of positions. Don't focus on getting a tight lock or a perfect lock; you are training your eyes to detect an *available* lock and your body to feel it.

You will also find as you increase the speed or if you gradually decide to increase the force that you learn a lot about what locks actually are, what it takes to make them work, and how to escape from them more efficiently. Remember that this drill is not a fight or a simulation. It is not about winning or losing. It is simply about learning to see and feel.

Immobilizations

> When someone wants to fight in an elevator, you push his face in to a corner. That simple. You don't give him the space to kick or throw an elbow. You keep your weight pressed into his back and he can't usually get the leverage to push away. Hell, if he does push away, you go with it and just pivot him face down to the ground.

Sometimes all you can do, or all you need to do, is to stop someone from moving. When we are talking immobilizations, we are not talking about sport pins or positions of dominance, but forcing the threat into a position where he cannot move and you can. Like locks, these are not fight-enders. These are techniques that you use to buy space or time to escape.

Immobilizations can be used to buy yourself a second to escape, to hold the threat until help can arrive, or to put him in a bad position so that you can use another technique. Oftentimes the follow up will have to be performed at a higher level of force, but not always.

Freezing the threat can be done with a tiny bit of effort, but it is not easy and takes good timing. The most common is pinning on the heels. When the weight is on both heels, right at the point of imbalance, the bad guy must recover his balance before he can move.

Humans are what a tracker would call a "direct register" animal. That means that when you are walking naturally, if your right foot is forward, your right hand is back. A sharp tug, straight down or slightly down and back, on the rear hand forces the center of gravity back and plants both feet. You can use the same technique with the back of the collar on a threat standing with his feet and shoulders square. If you watch American football, you have undoubtedly seen a horse-collar tackle, same principle with a twist at the end...

A threat can also be frozen in a state of unbalance. Bringing a threat up on his toes, or up onto his heels (subtly different than pinning on his heels), or posted on one foot prevents him from moving or striking effectively until he has recovered. This technique can buy you valuable time in a fight, and can also facilitate your ability to redirect or control an adversary.

The most common immobilization is to plant someone into a solid object—a wall, the hood of a car, the floor. There are a few tricks to making this more efficient. If his face is on the wall, the farther his feet are away from the wall, the less power he will have in trying to throw himself back. He, will, however, have a big triangle of space that he can use by collapsing or stepping in. Skilled opponents will escape that way. If he is pressed against the wall so that there's little to no space, on the other hand, he can apply much more power toward pushing himself off, and likely has the balance to kick backward or elbow effectively. Unless he is against the wall, his arms are not between him and the wall AND he is on his toes. Then he's pretty much screwed.

The best solution, often, is full length into the wall but up on his toes. You need to control both shoulders, probably with your forearm across his back, to prevent him from twisting.

It is okay to shove someone into a wall who is facing you, assuming all other justifications are in place. It is stupid to try to *immobilize* someone via wall or floor who is facing you. Immobilizing does not necessarily tie up arms or legs and puts you in prime striking range while keeping your own weapons busy. **Going for a face-up pin in a real fight is a sporting artifact that can get you killed.**

If the threat is this close in, this hands on, and especially if the threat takes you to the ground, this is not a polite game. The reason you can sometimes get away with a level of force as low as an immobilization is that you are not in danger of serious immediate injury. If you are in danger, use another technique. Escalate to the next level or even higher up as the situation warrants.

Even if you take someone to the ground face down, be careful about being tied up there. The situation can turn bad very quickly, particularly if the threat has friends nearby. If your goal is to escape, do so. The immobilization just buys you a second or two. You do not go all the way to the ground with the threat.

If you intend to hold the threat while help arrives (for instance a mentally ill child having a severe episode), be absolutely sure that you have enough of an edge in strength and skill to make it work. There can be an awful lot of pain and injury to hand out at that range. Be sure you need to do it and be sure you can handle it. And make sure there is no other threat that will put the boots to you while you're tied up.

There is a physiological lock that works on the ground with relatively low risk, although if the threat thrashes around enough he might injure himself. With the arm fully extended ninety degrees away from the body and the back of the elbow up, pressure just above the elbow can pin the whole body to the floor. The threat must be prevented from thrashing, particularly from moving the body closer to or away from the pinned arm. Nevertheless, this lock tends to be pretty reliable.

In real life, the winner in a ground fight is not the strongest, the meanest, or the most skillful. The winner will be decided by whose friends get there first.

Another technique that buys time, immobilizes the threat, and has minimal risk of injury is to step on the other guy's clothing when he is down. Baggy pants, in particular, immobilize both legs and the lower spine when you step on the saggy part just below the threat's crotch. Similarly, stepping on his collar with your foot inside his shirt can keep him from getting up and reengaging.

Some institutions, particularly those dealing with children, the mentally ill, and people in fragile health that are sometimes combative, advocate a "therapeutic hug" as a self-defense technique. At high levels of threat, particularly if weapons are involved, this policy is suicidal. At very low levels of threat, hugging someone until they calm down might work. It may also drive them into a panicked frenzy.

The key to making a "tactical hug" work is to control the elbows, knees, and head. You may still get pinched, but try to avoid bites, fingernail claws, and elbow or knee attacks. Possibly the best advantage of the hug is that if you are strong enough or in a good position, you can dump the threat on the ground and get away quickly.

Less impressive, but just as important, can be immobilizing a part of the threat. The elbow has enough leverage to control a threat's entire upper body. You can often control the legs with pressure on the shoulder. And there is always standing on a foot...

Elbow control works either through the crease of the elbow or the back of the elbow on the upper arm. A sudden grab thrust into the creases of both elbows freezes everything for a second. But just for a second, and you are in prime striking range. Unless you are better at wrestling, use the time to get out of there or transition to something else. And watch for head-butts.

The leverage point on the back of the elbow can be used to pull the threat off balance, turn him. Since we're talking about immobilizations, it is worth noting that you can place your body or even neck against the back of a threat's elbow to deny him the ability to turn or the distance he needs to develop sufficient power for an effective counterstrike.

There are limits, of course. Leverage increases power, but it isn't magic. The shoulders apply leverage across the spine and can affect the arms and the legs. If you apply force down on the threat's right shoulder, especially down and with a slight vector lateral to his body, that threatens his balance. And he cannot lift his right foot. A pull, twisting his right shoulder forward, can prevent him reaching you with his left foot or left fist. A little more force in any of these vectors can pull the threat off balance. Most people can't strike effectively when falling.

Pushing and Shoving (and Assisting)

We've more or less covered this in the projecting touch section already, but here is a bit more explanation. Pushing someone away can create space and time. In business, time is money. In a fight, time is safety. The threat must recover the distance, and that is one element of time. He will probably have to recover his balance and reorient as well. That's bonus time.

If a threat is pushing or charging, don't meet force with force. Unless the threat was stupid and decided, for some reason, to become aggressive with someone bigger and stronger, a strength contest with an adversary is a losing game. There are three principles that are critical for pushing someone who is bigger than you:

- Push from your strength into his weakness.
- Push with an upward vector.
- Exploit his momentum.

Push from your strength into his weakness

This may sound mystical, but it's just physics. No matter how you stand, your posture affects the directions you can move with power and the directions you can be easily unbalanced. If you stand with your feet together, you are vulnerable in every direction and cannot apply power. Any stance where your feet are farther apart than the length of your foot gives you a strong direction and a weak direction. The line from foot to foot is the strong direction. You can easily leap in that line. You can push.

A punch that ends directly in line with your strong line (or parallel to it) will have structure. A punch at an angle to that line will be weaker. A punch at right angles to the line is more likely to push you off balance than to hurt the threat. Perpendicular to that line and running right between the feet is the weak line. Use these stance variations to your advantage. If you push into the weak line, the threat is more likely to lose his balance.

Quick physics quiz—a strike into the strong line is apt to do more damage. Why?

Strong and weak lines are the grade-school explanation of what is going on here. But these descriptions are adequate for pushing people. So the first principle in pushing people is to push from your strong line into their weak line. Note that this is all about foot position. Hip and shoulder position are completely irrelevant. Unfortunately, most folks use hips and shoulders as a clue to where the feet are. That is wrong most of the time and is a specific reason why takedowns often fail. Force in the wrong direction is wasted.

Push with an upward vector

The second principle is to push with an upward vector. Not a lot; a very slight upward angle is enough. Pushing down can actually set the other guy on a firmer platform, keeping him from falling. Pushing straight across turns into a strength and weight contest; if you are the smaller combatant, you'll lose. A little upward vector breaks the threat's connection with the ground and makes everything more effective. It is also easier for short people, so take advantage of it.

Exploit his momentum

Exploiting momentum is a variation on the "gift" principle mentioned in the section "Joint Locks." If a threat is coming straight at you and you go straight at him, it will be a strength and weight contest. If you hit him at an angle, don't try to stop him but just make him miss; his own momentum, his own weight and speed become part of the force he must overcome to recover. Using the other guy's force against him is a time-honored strategy of the grappling arts. Time it well and you can be out of there by the time he turns around.

Pain

There wasn't much of a fight. The backup call came in and it was over before I could get through the four doors and up the stairs and sprint the 200 yards. One inmate, talking shit and making threats. He was already handcuffed. Four or five officers surrounding him, generally ignoring the rant, leading him off to disciplinary segregation.

As I got close, he made that distinctive hawking noise deep in his throat. I lunged forward, driving my thumb into the glands under the jaw, forcing his head to the side and up.

"Do NOT spit," I said. "I'm not sure I could save your life." It was also a felony. Spitting rarely ends well in corrections. Saliva is not a win-win.

"I wasn't gonna spit on *you,* sarge." As if who mattered.

Pain is unreliable and idiosyncratic. Some people curl up in a ball and start crying with a pinch. Other people—or even the exact same person on a different day—may not even feel a limb torn off in an accident. Endorphins? Sure. You don't think people get a boatload of endorphins when they fight?

When something worked really well in class, never forget that it worked on a healthy, sober, sane person who was not enraged, terrified, or drugged up.

Causing pain, especially in a survival fight, cannot be a primary goal. Sometimes it works, sometimes it does not; nevertheless, it almost always makes other techniques easier. Things work better, often, under the influence of a little pain.

And pain has one good side: **Pain is not injury.**

When you look at the force options, you see how important that concept is. The entire idea is to do the least harm to achieve the goal. It is best to have everything happen in the threat's own head. He sees a witness or a poor target choice and he moves on. Presence. Next best are a few words. It might hurt his feelings or disrupt his world view, but it does not even violate his personal space until we get to touch. Only at Level 4 do we make things happen or stop happening by pushing, pulling, locking, dropping, or pain. All of that is to avoid injury, and injury is the likely result of the strikes needed at Level 5. Level 5 is in preference to Level 6, which may leave not just a piece of meat who used to be a man, but possibly widows and orphans as well.

Pain is not injury. People who have not experienced much of either often confuse the two. Tasers and finger locks hurt, but they do far less injury than batons or fists. Screaming in pain makes for better video than swelling and discoloration and a joint that never works quite right again. People get outraged by the dramatic video and don't think of the real cost of the alternative. And then they sue… enough philosophy.

There are three legitimate reasons to use pain:

- As a bargaining tool. You jab a pressure point to say, "I will quit doing this if you will quit doing that." If the threat leaves, or lets go of the arm, the pain stops.
- To draw a response. It is still idiosyncratic, but lots of pressure points have fairly reliable flinches. If a grind across the ribs makes the threat jerk sideways, it can help throw him off when he is on top and you are on the ground, getting pounded. There

is a point under the jaw that tends to twist the spine up and back, setting up a sweep. An edge-of-hand "saw" across the jaw hinge tends to make people want to roll over into a better handcuffing position...you get the idea.

- To buy a second. A sudden, sharp, unexpected pain can be really distracting. Really bad pain, like some bites, can shut down the threat's brain for a short time and buy you an instant to do something else.

There is a fourth application for pain. It has no place in self-defense and, long-term, it is a loser but some people believe in education through pain. "I'm gonna teach you a lesson, boy." The challenge is that the lesson taught, when there is one, is almost never the lesson you think. If you get self-righteous and teach someone a lesson about using bad language in front of women, he does not learn to be more polite. He does learn that you're an insecure, power-tripping prick. That's lesson one. He will also learn that it is wiser to cause you harm from ambush next time, lesson two.

His third lesson is that you believe that power, the ability to beat him up, gives you the right to decide whom to beat up. He knows that you believe 'might makes right...and that may be okay with him. He may share that worldview. If he does, he may be compelled to "get his manhood back" by delivering a beating himself. Maybe to a woman or a child. And why not? You just sent the message loud and clear that he who can do it gets to decide.

You must be careful with any application of force, but pure pain has some special considerations. Using simultaneous multiple pressure points at one time seems to be less effective. We've found time and again that if multiple officers are all using pressure points, they seem to not work at all. Our working theory is that once the nerves get overloaded, the brain just quits registering them at all. Too much pain becomes noise and tends to be ignored.

Secondly, with pain or any of the techniques at Level 4, you are using a low level of force to deal with a relatively low level of threat. Constantly monitor the threat to ensure you are not driving them into a panic. Some people panic when held down. Some panic to pain. If the threat you are trying not to hurt suddenly goes into a fear-driven frenzy, someone may get hurt. Maybe you.

Hair

A very useful pain point that ordinary people think of but for some reason martial artists tend to forget about is hair. When it is available, a good fistful of head hair can be one of your most effective tools. It has the wonderful combination of pain *and* incredible leverage. Further, the leverage is applied to one of the most important control targets in the body—the spine.

It's easy to use if there is enough hair. Stick your fingers in, make a fist, give it a twist. Like any hold or lock, the technique must serve your goal. Twining your fingers in someone's hair doesn't exactly lend itself to running away.

The pain compliance aspect is pretty clear, but there are some nuances. Small amounts of hair hurt more than a fistful, but the grip is weaker. For most people, hair at the sides, just in front of the ear, seems to hurt more than other places on the head.

Used as a leverage application, always think in spirals. Oftentimes the leverage will be great enough that you can push, pull, bend or twist the threat's head, but not always. A strong neck can resist a lot of force. But it takes a much stronger neck to resist a force in multiple directions, such as a pull and a twist.

A spiral down and to the front makes the threat bend over, and can whip him off his feet. (Imagine you are standing face to face. Your right hand goes out, past the threat's head on his left side and then behind the head to grab the hair behind his right ear. Pull forward and down while twisting your hand palm up at your right hip.)

An upward spiral can pin him on his toes or heels or break his connection with the ground. If you can get his head moving fast enough, his feet will not be able to catch up and he will belly-plant onto the ground.

Hair techniques are not consequence free, nor are they completely safe. Slight variations on the torque can apply enough force to severely injure the neck, possibly resulting in paralysis or death (a much higher level of force). One of our mentors, after using a hair-hold to effect a takedown on a violent drunk later found a lock of hair with a piece of scalp still attached tangled in his fingers.

Pressure Points in General

There are all kinds of esoteric formulas out there designed to make pressure points work better. We are skeptical. We crunched the numbers on one of the more famous systems that describes times, cycles-of-destruction, polarities, and whatnot. We found that if the system is correct, it is impossible to survive a good massage. Here is a rule of thumb: If someone has to spend twenty minutes explaining what is supposed to happen before he tries it on you, the twenty-minute explanation is part of the technique. It may be it doesn't work so well under an instant assault.

Generally, you attack a pressure point with the smallest structured surface that you can. Finger or thumb tips work well, but it must be the tip (structured, bone) not the pad. The knuckles, the point of the elbow, even the forearm bones or shins can work. Some points work better pressed, some respond to a grinding action. All those particulars are covered for each individual point.

When you practice, you must use a partner and the partner must communicate. Digging in until he has deep bruises because the partner is too proud to say that you have done it right is not only stupid on the partner's side, but you do not learn anything either. Remember, this stuff doesn't work on everyone.

A note on pressure points, nerves, trigger points, and pain points: Purists get their panties in a twist on definitions. Which are nerve points? Which are meridians? What follows is a short list of relatively reliable points, what we have found them to do, and how to use them. The "why" and the definitions are window dressing. We're going for practical here.

You must be able to find the points, at the right angle, from different positions, with either hand (or other grinding surfaces) when you cannot see them. That is not so hard.

Specific Points

We once made a list of all the pressure points we have actually used and it ran to 113. Some are obscure (one on the chest that, for some reason, feels like burning for minutes after you stop applying pressure to it). Some are just wrong (sinus headache for a couple of days, anyone?). The points that follow are some of the more useful, as well as more consistently effective. Not all work on everybody, particularly if they are on certain drugs, enraged, or trained to "seal" them up. There are a few people who are insensitive to all or almost all pressure points. It has been said before and we'll say it again: If something does not work, do something else. Quickly.

Philtrum

The philtrum is the little divot in your upper lip right in the middle that runs from your lip to your nose. At the top of the philtrum, at the base of the nose, is a little ridge of bone. The rest of the nose is cartilage. Force applied inward and upward at the philtrum (think "extending the spine" not "squashing the skull") applies a lot of leverage on the head. And it hurts. A lot. Use the edge of your hand, taking care to keep the hand flat so it cannot be bit. This is the most reliable pain point we have found.

A great application for this is when two guys are wrestling around on the ground and you need to separate them. Step in from behind and use the philtrum to peel the guy on top off his victim. Another application is a standing come-along where you capture one arm, shoot your arm across the other guy's body, and use the blade edge of your hand to crank his head back at the philtrum. Keep the pressure on and you can usually move him with ease.

Mastoid

Taught at almost all police academies, the mastoid point is in the soft spot under the ear just behind the jaw. It hurts. Not everyone is sensitive to it, but if you press forward into the back of the jaw bone, instead of straight in, it tends to work better. This is a pure bargaining technique. The pain is not sharp enough to make a threat freeze, and the flinch is slow and not often useful. Most officers are taught to stabilize the head in any case.

Jaw hinge

Right at the muscles that bulges over the jaw.* You can deliver some pain by grounding with knuckles at this point while standing. The best applications for this point, however, are on the ground. If the threat is on his back, a grinding action over the point from the back toward his mouth makes him want to roll away. His face-down position is safer for you. The technique does not make him move, it just adds some influence. Forearm, shin, or even edge of the boot applied to the point when the threat is on the ground (face up or face down) makes him not want to move at all. A quick pressure here as you spring away buys you a little more time to leave.

Lymph nodes

In the soft spot right under the corner of the jaw is the same place your throat swells up when you are getting sick. A rigid thumb to this point, aimed like you are going right through the center of the skull, not only hurts but makes the head go back and up, exposing the throat, twisting the spine, and compromising balance. This application can be used to facilitate escalation to a higher level of force, say if the threat starts to draw a weapon.

Suprasternal notch

Is in the throat, right above the sternum, just below the cartilage of the trachea. Here is a big, stupid secret: Almost everything on the neck is a pressure point. You can pinch the muscles, squeeze the trachea, dig you fingers into the carotid triangle (if you're trying to be fancy), or pretty much any damn place and it all hurts. The thing about

* Important safety tip: Do NOT practice this technique on a partner who suffers from Temporal-Mandibular Joint Disorder (TMJ).

the suprasternal notch is that not only does it hurt, it also triggers the gag reflex. Most people back off when they are choking. The force is straight in on some people, or straight in and then down on others. This point does not work on everybody. A certain percentage of people do not have a gag reflex. This point becomes one of the least sensitive on the throat if you run into one of them. Can you say Plan B anyone…

Intercostals

Intercostals is a fancy way of saying the area between the ribs. Grinding your knuckles across the bones, right where the front and sides of the ribs make a "corner" makes some people flinch. It makes others squirm. It's amazing how many big, macho, martial artists and cops are really ticklish. Most people find it unpleasant (not agonizing) and turn away from the sensation.

Axillary

Axillary is the medical term for the armpit. If you can get a stiffened finger or two deep into the armpit, go deep, right between the muscles until you feel bone, it hurts quite a lot. Most people jerk away and try to clamp their arm down, which can shorten their reach and make them let go of things (like weapons they might wish to draw or deploy). Easier to reach and sometimes just as useful, if you have strong fingers, is digging into either the pectoral or trapezius muscles that frame the armpit.

Inguinal

Inguinal is the crease where the thigh meets the body in front. It is the same place where first aid class teaches you to put pressure on the femoral artery to slow bleeding. It feels icky. It hurts a little, tends to make that hip flinch back, compromising structure, and it makes a lot of people feel violated.

Triceps tendon

Located directly on the back of the upper arm about an inch above the elbow, this tendon is only accessible if the arm is straight. Using this point makes all of the armbars work better. When standing, pain is best achieved when standing, with a grind or rub across the back of the arm. On the ground, however, once the threat is face down and the arm extended to the side (see the physiological lock under in the "Immobilizations" section above), you can kneel or even stand on this point. If the threat can feel pain at all, this application will usually make him not want to fight.

Inner elbow

There are actually a suite of four effective pressure points on the inner elbow, two on the upper arm and two on the forearm. The most useful is on the thumb side, just below the crease of the elbow, right at the top of that little muscle mound. When the elbow is bent, it already makes a good leverage point to twist the threat's body. The pressure point adds a little emphasis.

Inner thigh

On the inside of the upper leg about two or three inches above the knee is a remarkably sensitive spot. It is vulnerable to a swift toe-kick, particularly if you are wearing boots. A strike there can make the leg wobble or collapse. This technique is often used in sports martial arts as a way to break out of a guard, by pressing your elbows into both of the opponent's pressure points at the same time. The point tends to make the legs pop apart. You can also stand on this pressure point while controlling the threat's opposite leg in an Achilles lock.

Side of knee

There are several pressure points on the foot and leg, but most are not really helpful in a self-defense situation. Some points are better kicked or kneed (Level 5) than used purely for pain or control. The best pure pain point is on the outside of the leg and slightly back, below the knee and just under the bony knob. It hurts if pressed or ground, but it is most useful for making someone stay down once they are on the ground or pushing away as you escape.

Takedowns

He was bare-chested, remnants of purple and gold body-paint clinging to his skin. It looked like there'd been a letter written on his chest, but the frigid downpour had washed most of it off. I would have thought he'd be cold, running around with no shirt in all that rain, but he didn't seem to notice. Probably because he was working himself into a rage.

Unfortunately, the object of that all anger was my employee, a young woman a full head shorter and a good hundred pounds lighter than the threat. They were standing next to the chain-link fence, where a gate allowed access to the football field. Cussing, spitting, gesticulating wildly, he was right up in her face. She held her ground, but I was afraid she was about to get hurt.

"I'll fucking go where I want to go, bitch. I want on the field and you can't stop me!"

As I approached his blind side, he shoved his hand into her face, two fingers pressing up against her nose. He'd touched her. I could act.

I reached across, grabbed his hand, cranked his wrist, and pivoted in a sharp spiral. From the shocked expression on his face, he hadn't even realized that I was there. Then he landed in a mud puddle with a satisfying splash. I kept a hold of his wrist, planted a foot on his upper arm at the shoulder, and held him there until an officer arrived.

He blew a blood alcohol level of 0.13. That's one hell of a tolerance for a nineteen-year-old.

Getting a threat off his feet will rely on many of the principles already discussed, particularly gifts and maximizing leverage. Your ability to apply a throw or sweep in a struggle is heavily influenced by how you practice. In order to improvise under pressure, just going through the motions will not be enough. You must practice with live, moving, resisting opponents.

That said, you will develop bad habits and waste much time. Judoka become so good at throwing because they work against people who are specifically resisting throws. That's good, except one of the most common ways in real life to resist a throw is to punch you in the nose. Judoka don't regularly practice against that.

It is also far, far easier to get a throw in real life than in a competition. In competition, in order to get a shoulder or full-entry hip throw, you must use exquisite timing and explosive movement to get your back to the opponent without him exploiting your vulnerability.

In real life, you will get the same throw because the threat grabbed you from behind. The hard part in competition is often the easy part in real life. Not exactly what you'd expect, but true.

Like any aspect of grappling or close-range fighting, just reading a book or article is a terrible way to develop the skill. Grappling is profoundly tactile. You must feel in order to understand. You must feel it moving and in chaos before you can really use it. Find a good instructor and spend some time on the mat.

Balance

There are thousands upon thousands of throws, but in the end there are only a very few ways to get someone on the ground without injuring them. Now it is time for that more advanced way to look at balance.

It's not just lines. Your feet make a base. In grappling, every point of contact you have with the ground helps create stability. Just like the base on a chess piece. If you are standing with feet shoulder width apart, the base can be outlined as the outside edge of your feet, a line toe to toe, and another line heel to heel, making a rectangle. A similar base can be drawn for any foot configuration or body position on the ground.

About a hand's breadth below the navel and halfway between your belly and your spine is your Center of Gravity (CoG). If your center of gravity leaves your base, you lose balance. If you do not get your base under it quickly, you fall. That is all falling really is.

From this perspective, the weak lines of balance are merely the places where the CoG is closest to the edge of the base. The strong lines are strong because you would have to move the CoG farther to get the same effect. From this model, you can see that you affect a takedown by moving the CoG outside of the base, by changing the shape of the base so that the CoG is no longer supported, or by damaging the structure supporting the CoG.

That probably seems kind of convoluted, but it is simple. Understanding something simply really helps when you need to improvise under pressure.

What follows are some types of takedowns. In real life, there are a lot of mixed types. It is more efficient to add good leverage and a sweep to the threat's momentum than to use any of the three ideas alone. The classifications help explain the concept, nothing more.

Momentum takedowns

Sometimes when the threat is putting a lot of energy into an action, like a powerful swing, a kick, or a charge, his CoG will outrun his base. Or his base will outrun his CoG as in a kick, à la Charlie Brown going after the football when it is suddenly pulled away. If there is enough power, you simply get out of his way.

Sometimes a little steering is necessary in order to keep the center of gravity moving. The judo throw *uke otoshi* is based on *uke* (the opponent) taking a powerful step and *tori* (that'd be you) tugging slightly, keeping the CoG moving straight over the forward foot. The back foot cannot move up to catch the balance. *Uke* falls down.

Sometimes, as in curling up into a turtle when being chased, the feet are blocked to prevent them from catching the CoG. Same result. Bad guy falls down, goes boom.

Leverage takedowns

When you just push someone over, it is often leverage: pushing on the chin while stabilizing the spine, or the head and arm throw. Even *osoto-gari*, the outside leg sweep, uses leverage so effectively that often the sweeping action is unnecessary. That is particularly true when you corkscrew the adversary rather than pulling straight or at an angle.

Sweeps

Sweeps are simple. Sort of. There are several categories.

In a *static sweep*, you freeze the threat's center of gravity over one side of his base and then knock the support leg out from under that side. Simple. The outer reap (e.g., *osoto gari*) is the most common example. You must pin the weight over the foot. This sweep fails if you attempt it on a foot that is in the air because the center of gravity is over the other foot.

Other sweeps are *moving sweeps*. The act of walking (or running or combat footwork) involves shifting your center of gravity outside of your base as you change the base to catch it. That sounds complicated, but it is only this: Walking is merely a controlled falling. Each step is catching your balance with a new base before you can finish the fall. You move forward.

In a moving sweep, you prevent the foot from catching the center of gravity. To pull off a moving sweep in a competition requires exquisite timing, even more so in a serious fight. It can be fairly easy trying to apply to a slow drunk whom you do not want to hurt but do need to stop. The cool thing about moving sweeps is that if you have exquisite timing; they require almost no strength. The threat practically throws himself.

You must sweep the foot that is about to catch the weight and do it before the foot actually touches the ground. Executing your move before the threat's foot touches down is the key to timing any moving sweep.

A note on technique and techniques: There are lots of different throws, sweeps, and takedowns in martial arts. You can memorize a whole bunch or you can learn the principles, learn to recognize the opportunity (gifts), and improvise. *Osoto gari* sweeps the entire length of the opponent's leg. *Osoto gake* chops at his ankle. From a principles-based standpoint, the difference is cosmetic. You are removing one of the props that he needs for balance, the specific prop he is most committed to. Whether you remove that prop with the whole length of your leg, a powerful kick, or a chainsaw, the effect is the same, although a chainsaw would be considered a much higher level of force.

You can stop the foot, as in a classic *sasae tsurikomi ashi* (lifting, pulling foot sweep): as the threat steps forward, his back foot must become his front foot. This motion is commonly called taking a step. You put something in the way of that (your own foot, the tip of a cane, or a low obstacle you can kick), the threat falls. Ever missed a step? Tripping, is what we call it when it happens by accident. If you are behind the threat and have good timing, you can knock his advancing foot sideways across his centerline so that it catches on the back of his own leg. Tripping over his own feet.

You can also cross the foot, as in *de ashi harai* (single-foot sweep). The advancing foot gets kicked or gently guided across the threat's centerline. The step never gets under the center of gravity.

You can also extend a moving sweep. The foot advances and you keep pulling it forward, never letting it touch the ground, à la *ko uchi gari* (minor inner foot reap). The threat's sensation is that he took a step that just kept getting longer and longer without ever touching the ground. He threw his foot at the floor and missed. If he could do it with his whole body, it would be flight. Do it with just part of the body and it is falling.

From the principles of base and CoG, it should be obvious why there is no judo sweep that spreads the legs to the outside. (We keep kicking these little things to you, like "it should be obvious" or "explain why" or throw out a question without an answer. This is *important*. You need to think for yourself. Always. You need to understand stuff, not just know it. Everything in this or any book is just words on a page. That's, at best, knowledge. You want to apply this when you are scared and desperate, so you need, at minimum, understanding. When you can tie things together, draw conclusions, and see connections, you are at least moving in the right direction.)

True throws

Yeah, I love judo. So? What I classify as true throws are techniques where you get your center of gravity under the threat's CoG and break his connection with the ground. Then you follow through.

Often by spinning him over your CoG, but sometimes just by hip-bumping high enough that his legs get in the air and guiding his upper body to hit first.

You must be close to make classical throws work. We do not hold backpacks away from our backs. When you slam a car door with a quick hip action because your hands are full, you can't do it at a distance. This is body-contact stuff.

Throws, in real life, are often easy if you get the right gift. When grabbed tight from behind by a taller person, the set-up is natural. You must, however, learn to maintain or recover your spine integrity in order to pull the throw off. If the other guy grabs you from behind in such a way that you are straight-backed, especially on your toes and leaning back, you will not be able to apply force. Your straightened or concave spine robs your abdominal muscles and legs of power.

There are two ways to recover:

- The butt slam, where you thrust your pelvis forward to create space, and then slam your butt backward into the threat's groin.
- Going limp, which often creates a throw all by itself.

Bonus point: If you drop suddenly so that you are on one knee, the down leg hooking the threat's foot, you have combined a true throw with a momentum ploy with a moving/stop sweep. See how this works?

When in a scuffle (We chose this word carefully; in a real survival fight, throws are extras. You need to concentrate on damage. Sure, the ground can hit harder than the fist, but only if the other guy doesn't know how to fall properly. There are an awful lot of experienced grapplers out there...), clinches of various types are common. Many people try to hold their hips back in a clinch, which makes them extremely vulnerable to the class of forced-momentum throws called sacrifice throws or *sutemi-waza*. Holding your hips back, especially if the clinch angles off to the side such as when the other guy is looking for a headlock, often gives you exactly what you need to slip your hip in low to his front and do one of the classic hip throws.

One of the easiest of the true throws is to come up behind the threat, grab him tight with your own CoG low, and thrust your hips forward while straightening your legs. Your CoG will make a wave action under his CoG and knock his feet high in the air.

That's all cool about getting the threat into the air. You also have to talk about the ground. Throws end when the unfortunate recipient stops falling, not when he starts falling. Abrasions and minor bruising are the most common injuries from takedowns. Someone thrown into a table or the edge of a curb, however, could be seriously injured. By serious, we mean broken spine. Back of the head caved in. Stuff like that. If deadly force is justified, that is not an issue. If it is not (and remember we are talking Level 4 here), doing it deliberately is excessive force

Doing this type of takedown by accident would be tragic—picture this: *You're in a play scuffle with your best friend. He's been drinking and wants to drive home. You want him to wait a bit. You're buddies, so the mild argument turns into playful pushing. You want to show him he's too drunk to be coordinated so you effortlessly trip him—and he hits the edge of the coffee table going down. He can't feel his feet…*

That is not intended to discourage you. If a takedown is appropriate, use a takedown. Just as there is no technique that works every time, there is no technique that is 100 percent safe, either. Rory once put a finger-lock on a guy in a Norse-wrestling competition and he went completely berserk. How was he to know that a 300-pound-biker-looking dude was a concert cellist?

If you are in excellent control of the situation, you can literally guide the fall. If appropriate, slow the descent and let or make the threat spread out on the surface area or even roll with the impact. The follow-through commonly taught with the true throws (judo hip and shoulder throws) is specifically designed to minimize injury. Pulling up on the arm at the last minute may give you opportunities to apply pins and locks, but the real purpose is to minimize injury. You do not see that movement in *koryu* forms, the battlefield martial arts.

These older systems had follow-throughs that were designed to cause damage by:

- Focusing impact on the cervical spine (potentially lethal).
- Targeting the point of the shoulder (crippling).
- Attacking the tailbone, which hurts unbelievably, but you get over it (is there a word for short-term crippling?).
- Knocking the wind out of the adversary (temporary incapacitation).

That is without deliberately aiming at sharp corners, traffic, or big drop-offs, any of which can significantly increase the amount of damage the victim receives from the throw itself. As you can see, they didn't mess around in the *koryu* martial arts.

Knee pops

Knee pops are a nice way to destroy the structure that supports the center of gravity. Obviously a straight knee can be popped forward with a light kick, but there are several "pops" that work well in extremely close fights.

A straight knee is vulnerable from all four sides. Sharp pressure or a blow on the side or front of a knee can cause permanent injury. A bent knee is vulnerable from the sides and somewhat from the back. The side pops from the inside can cause injury if done sharply, but if done a little slower, the knee has a tendency to "give," jerking away from the force, opening the hips, and compromising structure. Side pops on the outside of a bent knee tend to turn the knee across the centerline, usually compromising balance and often giving you the threat's back. Turn him so that you can strike from behind where he cannot defend himself. There are two ways of getting behind someone, moving you or moving him. Moving him is better, albeit harder to pull off most of the time.

To pop into the back of a bent knee, you go up on your toes so that your knee is above his and press in and down at the pressure point just below the knee. The calf muscle separates near the top of the fibula into two heads (that is the technical term—biceps means "two heads," triceps means "three heads"). You press directly between them, in and down. This technique sometimes has the wonderful effect of leaving a threat on his knees with his back to you. That is about as good as it gets if you want to neutralize a threat without injury.

To practice knee pops, work from a tight clinch. The partner practicing raises one foot up on the ball of the foot. This motion gives elevation and reach. Because the foot does not leave the ground, it preserves balance and is much harder to feel coming than any technique where the foot does leave the ground.

From that lifted position, the partner feels for what he can reach on his partner's knees, whether they can be knocked from inside, outside, or pressed into the front.

Lock Takedowns

If you have a strong lock, you can force a threat down by pressing the lock into the ground, as in an armbar takedown. Alternatively, by creating a big motion and applying the force in the lock upward, you can break the threat's connection with the ground.

Locking upward works better on trained martial artists. Many have been conditioned to go with the lock and wind up throwing themselves. Untrained people may well be injured if you apply enough force to a joint to lift them into the air.

Using Level 4 Techniques at Higher Levels of Force

Level 4 techniques work by making the threat not want to fight. They are largely psychological. If it hurts enough, he may decide to go home. If he must pick himself up off the ground, he may decide that there is more to his victim than he thought and go elsewhere. If the bad guy finds himself unable to move, even for a second, he may change his mind and reassess his goals.

Level 4 is all about the mind.

If someone wants to kill, rape, or maim you, changing his mind is not enough. It might be, maybe, but you cannot read his mind. If someone tries to stab you and misses, then apologizes, is he now safe?

What if wants to shake your hand? While still holding the knife?

If a threat is bent on your destruction, you need to take away his means or opportunity or both. You take away opportunity by escaping. **You take away means by breaking him.** Re-read that sentence. You take away a threat's means to cause you harm by breaking the threat.

If you could escape, you would not be going hands on. Keep an eye out for the opportunity, but if you cannot escape a serious assault, you must concentrate on breaking the threat.

The Level 4 techniques aren't very good at that. Some, particularly the locks and the takedowns, can do significant damage. These techniques require pretty specific gifts. They can be relatively difficult and intricate to pull off, and they might tie up more of your resources (e.g., using both of your hands in an attempt to control one of the threat's) than you can afford.

All true, but if the gift presents itself, go for it. Don't get so caught up in trying to punch, kick, and bite your way out of the corner that you miss the opportunity to slam a straight elbow into a doorjamb. If you can knock the guy down, it could be exactly what you need to escape. If he must get up before attacking you, it buys you time to run.

Pop quiz time: If you study an art that has takedowns and you have a favorite, dissect it. What combination of true throw, momentum, leverage, lock, sweep, or whatever is your favorite? Whether it's *irimi nage* clothesline, double-leg, or other takedown, what is your "go to" application? How does it work? Now, look at it again. Can you refine a piece of the technique to make it more street effective? For example, *osoto-gari* leg sweeps work even better when you push on (or strike) the other guy's chin, increasing the leverage aspect. Can you add a piece entirely to improve upon it? For example, it is completely against the rules for most any competition, but sometimes when you are being forced into the concrete anyway, you can modify a shoot to snap the threat's knee to the outside, adding a lock component to a technique that is already effective. Finally, what is your bail-out strategy if it doesn't work?

There is the added bonus as well that if you can justify deadly force and you managed to resolve it at Level 4, you have a very, very good case that you were the good guy.

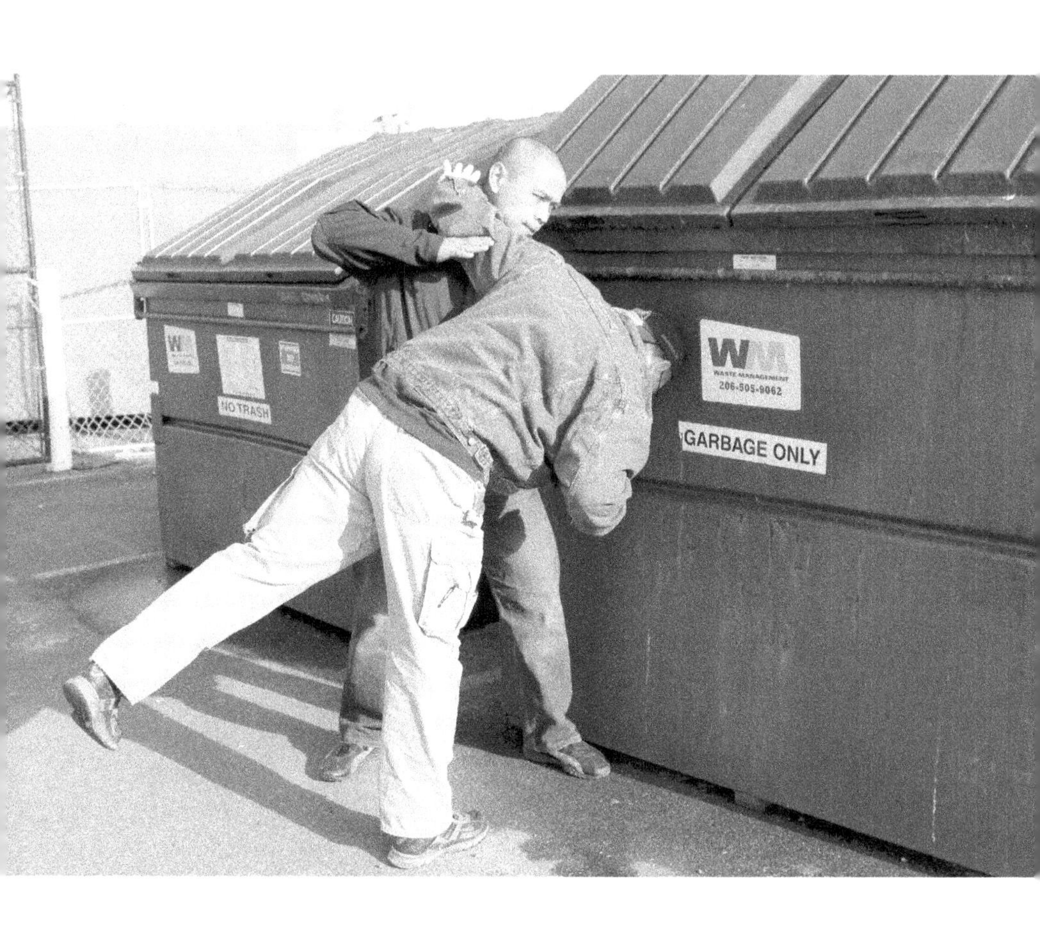
WM
WASTE MANAGEMENT
206-505-9062
GARBAGE ONLY
NO TRASH

INTERLUDE—THE 4/5 SPLIT

Here is something that you need to grasp at a very deep level. However you look at it, all the problems you can deal with at Level 1 through Level 4 belong in one world. You cross that line to Level 5 and it is an entirely different world.

You can break it up in many ways:

- At Level 4 and below, you are trying *not* to injure the threat. At Level 5, injuring the threat so that he cannot harm you is your first priority.
- You use Level 4 and below when you are in control. You escalate to Level 5 when the threat is in control.
- If you are trying to control behavior, you are at Level 4 and below. When you are trying to control incoming damage, you are at Level 5.
- Level 1 up to Level 4 are appropriate when the stakes are low. When the stakes become your health or life, you must be working at Level 5 or 6.
- You use up to Level 4 when you are winning. When you are losing, you need to be at Level 5.

This list can go on... "Position before submission" is not a winning strategy; it is a winner's strategy. When you have the edge in skill and conditioning, when you are winning, you want to consolidate your position and try to limit surprises. When you are losing, you want to introduce enough chaos to maybe break an opportunity loose for a successful counterattack. If you are losing the grappling match, it may behoove you to turn it into a knife fight. (Pop quiz: How would you justify that in court?)

As we escalate to Level 5, be aware that the fight has now become about damage. It is a different world and requires a different mindset. **You will not get to choose Level 5. It will be thrust upon you.**

If you have time to think, "I don't think I can wrestle this guy. I'd better get a baseball bat," you are contemplating assault. If you have time to think and plan and marshal resources, you should be able to come up with something that works from a lower, not a higher level of force.

If you suddenly find your head slammed into a wall and something jamming into your kidneys, and you're hoping it is just a fist and not a knife—well, you need to use as much force as you need to get out alive. You need to use as much force as you can.

As a law-abiding citizen, you do not pick Level 5. If you find yourself at Level 5 or 6, you had no choice.

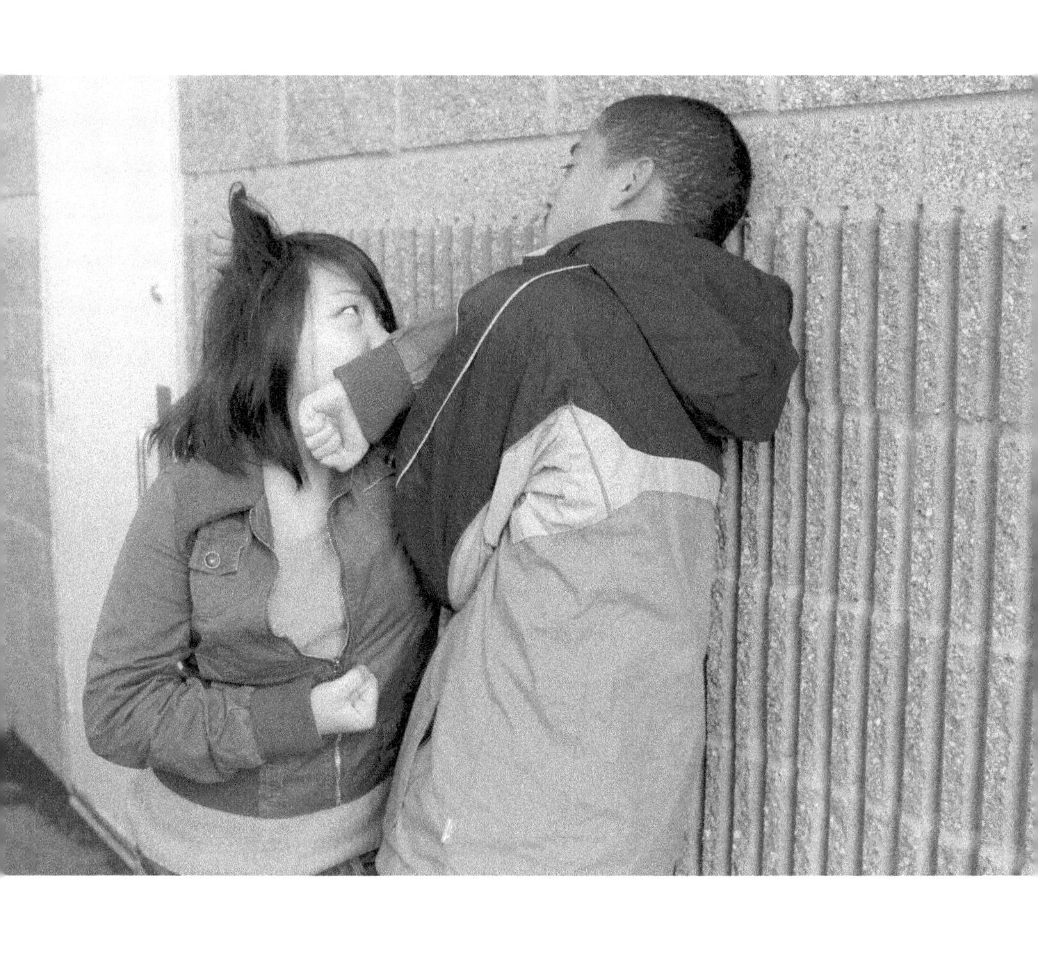

LEVEL 5—LESS-LETHAL FORCE

Welcome to Level 5. Here, you are committing a crime. It doesn't matter whether you are actually charged with one or not, Level 5 is a crime. If you're a black belt or ranked tournament competitor, it's pretty easy for the district attorney to find out via a quick Google search. In most jurisdictions, "trained fighters" are held to a higher standard than regular folks when it comes to prosecuting violence, so you really need to watch yourself if you're in this category.

At best it is a simple assault, but if things go awry it could be anything from aggravated assault to manslaughter to murder. If intent, means, opportunity, and preclusion are there, with a good lawyer, a *lot* of money, and a little luck, you will be off the hook because the actions you took outweigh the competing harm of what the other guy was going to do to you. As mentioned previously, self-defense is an affirmative plea; you admit to the crime and then need to prove you had a good reason not to be held accountable.

Level 5 is about damaging the other guy, typically so that you can withdraw and flee to safety. Consequently, less-lethal force tends to be delivered via striking techniques. While there are a limited number of striking elements such as elbows, knees, hands, feet, forearms, shins, and head, targeting makes a significant difference in the level of force applied. A punch to the ribs for example may cause damage, but the effect is largely psychological when it comes to ending a fight. The exact same punch to the jaw hinge, on the other hand, could cause loss of consciousness. Location matters.

Most fights end when one guy or the other gives up, rather than when he can no longer continue to battle. In a fistfight, it is tough to do enough physiological damage to kill or severely disable someone. If you watch MMA competitions, for example, you will see competitors who have been kicked or kneed in the head continue to fight, and those who are knocked out virtually always walk away from the ring under their own power afterward. The psychological damage from a broken bone will take many people out of a fight. Many, but by no means all... "Knockout" blows don't always work.

The goal of less-lethal force is to stop an attacker and facilitate your escape to safety without permanently injuring or killing him. Sometimes you hit him. Sometimes you knock him into something that can cause pain or injury. Or use an implement to whack him with. Nevertheless, the things you do in this category should be less likely to cause lethal damage or permanent injury than actions taken at the next level on the force continuum. This goal generally means employing empty-hand techniques designed to incapacitate or using tools such as pepper spray or Tasers that are designed to be less than lethal.

"Less-lethal" weapons are explicitly designed and primarily employed to incapacitate people, while minimizing fatalities, permanent injury, and damage to property or the environment. These weapons include devices such as Tasers or OC (Oleoresin Capsicum or "pepper") spray that are employed by civilians and law enforcement officers alike (though civilians have fewer options to choose from). Simply because these items are designed to be non-lethal does not mean that they have a zero probability of maiming or killing someone.

It is not just what you use, but how you use it. Knocking the other guy onto a piece of furniture often plays better in court than smacking him over the head with a chair, for example, even though you can do similar damage either way.

Other types of weapons that could be used in less than lethal ways are often seen as a higher level of force when adjudicated by the courts. Even the tactical baton,

Strictly speaking, Tasers and OC are pain compliance tools, Level 4. Pepper spray is an irritant. Fifteen minutes or so of cold water or forty-five minutes in a breeze and your eyes might still be red but everything is fine. Once the Taser is done cycling, you have two barbed needles in you, roughly the equivalent of getting a fishhook in your thumb. Neither tool does enough physical damage to stop anyone.

However, there is a perception that any tool, even a tool designed to do NO physiological damage is a higher level of force than an unarmed technique that is readily capable of damage, like a jointlock. That perception, which is something you can expect from a jury or a prosecutor, is why we chose to classify these tools at Level 5 for the purpose of this book.

which is not even designated as a deadly weapon some places, tends to be held to that standard more often than not when deployed by a civilian because of the damage it *could* do, not necessarily because of the damage it does when you use it. In certain instances, you may be judged by the target (e.g., leg versus head) when the prosecutor decides which charges to bring, but you probably shouldn't count on that.

Use of an implement explicitly designed as a weapon raises the stakes even further. For example, a knife is a tool, but in most jurisdictions it is designated a deadly weapon. Consequently, while you could use an unopened folding knife for control techniques, in most jurisdictions you will be charged with the aggravated assault (or attempted murder), just like you would be if you had opened the blade. Similarly, you could use a firearm to leverage an armbar, but that'd be stupid. Because you should plan on having to justify its use as Level 6, we will take the conservative route and cover these types of weapons in the next section.

Hitting Hard

If you are going to damage someone, you will need to hit hard to do it. Or use a tool. We will assume that if you are studying some type of martial art, you will become proficient with the tactics and techniques of your style. Consequently, we are not going to delve too deeply into the mechanics of striking. You can't master this stuff from a book anyway. Nevertheless, there are a few principles that are worth relating that apply to most any fighting method.

Stay connected

Be it a kick or a punch, body alignment is the key to hitting hard. The more connected your striking appendage is to your body, the more energy is transferred into the target. That is why a straight punch that lands with the elbow down, shoulder relaxed, spine straight, and deltoid muscles locked down tight hurts more than an identical punch where the elbow is raised a bit. Every joint has a potential for a disconnect. This disconnectedness breaks the "power chain," allowing energy to bleed off. You are hitting with your arm rather than with your full body weight. Don't break the power chain.

Use your core

Try this with a partner: Shake hands. Using your forearm, you will see that you only move his forearm. If you use your shoulder, however, you can move his whole arm. If you use your hip, so that your whole body is engaged, you can move his core. Tying with the previous principle, a connected power chain helps you put your entire body weight behind your blows so that nothing bleeds off when you strike from you core.

Accelerate

Acceleration is critical too. If the speed remains constant, you are pushing the other guy; whereas if your blow lands faster than it started, you are striking. You can strike much faster if you relax until the moment your fist (or foot or whatever) hits the target and then tense your whole body than you can if you remain tense the entire time. Actually, with good bone to bone structure, the tensing is unnecessary and slows down your recovery, but that requires a lot of skill to apply. Weight drops add additional force too.

Practice

Staying connected using your core and accelerating into your target will markedly increase your effectiveness, but you need to practice in order to make it work reliably. Practicing with a heavy bag or *makiwara* (striking post) can help you build and refine these fundamentals of striking. Simply pressing against a solid object and feeling your body alignment helps. Specialized Body Opponent Bags (BOBs) help with targeting too. The BOB is shaped like the torso and head of real person. There are also extended models that include the groin. BOB facilitates contouring strikes to various vital points such as the eyes, and is soft enough to strike hard without damaging your hands, assuming you do it correctly.

Drills with striking pads or shields will help you move from static to dynamic positioning and help you adjust to different ranges. In a fight, you can bet your target will be moving. You must practice delivering effective power to a moving target. This type of practice is very useful because unlike sparring, you can go full out without endangering your training partner. Do work up to it slowly under proper supervision so that you don't hurt yourself.

Hand Techniques

Martial artists learn dozens of striking techniques with their hands. Some relate to the position of the fist and rotation of the arm when it connects with the adversary, such as an uppercut, standing fist, or fore-fist punch, all of which can be found in the classical karate "corkscrew." Others relate to the part of the hand that you strike with your opponent with, such as hammerfist, palm heel, knuckles, or fingers. Others yet relate to the trajectory that the punch follows to its target, such as a swing strike, straight punch, or hook.

Open-hand techniques can be safer to perform than closed hand ones on the street, as Mike Tyson discovered the hard way when he broke his hand punching fellow boxer Mitch Green in a bar fight in 1988. Unless you are a very experienced martial artist, it is best to stay away from most closed-fisted techniques, save for the hammerfist where you are hitting with the side of your hand. Oftentimes a palm-heel or other open-hand strike is as effective as and much safer than hitting with your knuckles.

If you are skilled enough to strike with a closed hand, be sure to connect with the first two knuckles (base of your index and middle finger) rather than the last two. This connection aligns the hand with the arm properly and is much less likely to result in debilitating injury if you hit the wrong target. Boxers, MMA competitors, and others who practice with gloves often hit improperly and injure themselves in street fights. Regardless, closed fists that are seen by witnesses, or more importantly captured on film, do not play as well in front of a jury as open hands do, despite the fact that skilled practitioners can cause serious injury either way. Even though millions of people spend at least a little time in a *dojo*, often in their youth, most jurors' "experience" with fighting in general and martial arts in particular stems from Hollywood movies, not real life experience. This can be a real challenge in court.

You can also strike with your elbow or forearm. These are very effective striking surfaces if you have limited experience because you can hit hard with somewhat less risk of injuring yourself than using your hand. Examine your art; many so-called "blocks" are actually forearm strikes when performed properly.

Foot Techniques

Kicks begin by forcefully lifting the knee as quickly as possible. If the adversary is close enough, this movement becomes the initial strike. Depending on where you aim and your proximity to the other guy, it is possible to strike with the knee and leg or foot all with the same motion, connecting multiple times. The higher you lift your knee, within reason, the better. Like a punch, the foot should be moving faster when it lands than when it begins or it will wind up being more of a push than a strike. Pushes can be useful, but they rarely cause damage (unless the other guy stumbles into or lands on something that hurts him).

After the knee lift, you can perform different kicks by varying what the rest of your leg does. For example, to do a front kick, swing your foot up, snap it forward, and bring it back as quickly as possible (sorta like trying to kick your own butt on the return motion). For a stomp kick, drive your foot downward leading with your heel. To do a sidekick, rotate your hip and snap the kick out to the side. Front kicks, stomps, and sidekicks are generally the easiest kicks to learn, although fancier applications like axe kicks have their place as well. Having said that, however, if you are going to kick an adversary in a fight, the safest place to aim is below his waist. Low kicks are faster, more direct, and harder to block than high ones. They also help you retain your balance.

While many martial artists train barefoot, your feet are much more likely than not to be shod if you get into a real fight. That means your boot or shoe can become a weapon. Or it can blunt some of the force of the blow. Certain types of footwear make great striking surfaces (for example, steel-toed boot), and they protect your foot too.

Be sure to practice kicking in shoes. This could damage a BOB or heavy bag, so you might consider using a fencepost, *makiwara*, or even a wall. Start with low power and gradually build up. As you do, practice using the shoe in a way that does not injure your foot. You will find quickly that with soft shoes, like most athletic trainers, you will want to curl your toes back much like a traditional barefoot strike. With hard-soled shoes, like dress shoes or boots, you will find that pressing your toes hard against the sole allows you to use the point of the sole as a striking surface, like kicking with a board.

Assaults happen at a much closer range than most people practice sparring. This distance especially affects kicks. Whether kicking above the waist is a good tactic is one question. The simple fact is that in most assaults, you won't have the room.

We will do variations on this exercise a couple of times: Go hit a heavy bag as hard and fast as you can. Flurry on it for maximum damage, the same way a predator would try to take you out. Then let the bag dangle and see how close you are. That is the range where your techniques need to work. Toe kicking the ankle is one of the best techniques simply because there often is not room for anything else.

Contouring

Contouring is a very important component of fighting, yet it is commonly overlooked because it becomes pretty much irrelevant in tournament competitions where safety gear and heavy gloves change the dynamics. Contouring helps you identify the best target for any given technique, assuring that you do maximum damage to the adversary and minimize the risk of injury to yourself. In general, hard parts strike soft targets and vice versa.

If you have ever punched someone in the jaw with your closed fist, you undoubtedly know how painful that can be for both parties. Hard fist to hard jaw is not good. A palm-heel strike to the jaw, on the other hand, can be quite effective. Soft palm to hard jaw works. It not only meets the contouring rule, but it is far more painful for the other guy.

If you take a close look at all of your striking surfaces, your feet, hands, knees, and elbows, you can see how targeting works at a more granular level. For example, a single knuckle or finger strike fits the solar plexus better than the whole fist, even when you make it properly by connecting solely with the first two knuckles. A hammerfist aligns much better with the temple or the forehead than it does with the stomach where an uppercut or palm-up straight punch might better apply. A bear claw (second knuckle of all four fingers) or web hand (between the thumb and index finger) can strike the throat, whereas a palm heel simply will not fit.

The same approach works with your feet too. Even when shod, the blade edge of your foot aligns best with the other guy's knee, while the ball of your foot makes a good fit with his groin or midsection, particularly if you use an upward arc when you strike. Alignment of the foot matters too; the heel works better for a stomp or back kick than it does for a front kick. As you can see, different types of kicks are best for different targets.

Making It Work When You Are Losing

Okay, so you know how to hit hard. Most martial artists do. The challenge in a Level 5 (or Level 6) encounter is that unless you are the attacker, odds are good that you are losing. If you were winning, you would not need to take things to Level 5. And that's the real bitch. Losing in an assault is not like losing at sparring or *randori*, no matter how intense the match.

This simple fact is where so much self-defense advice falls apart.

What does it feel like to be on the losing end of an assault? Everything is wrong. The bad guy set it up for you to be at a disadvantage. The action will be too close, too fast. Pain and damage will be coming in. Totally untrained people hit four times a second. An experienced violent criminal, unarmed, will likely hit you four times before your brain can switch from whatever you were thinking about before to your fighting mode.

If the threat is armed, the speed does not change. The damage just increases.

Experienced criminals will hamper your mobility. The attack will be close. Try this: Go to a heavy bag and set an alarm or get someone to blow a whistle. Relax. When the whistle blows, unload on the heavy bag as fast and hard as you can. Have the whistle blow again in three seconds. Freeze. Let the bag hang.

When the bag hangs, it is probably touching you. Maybe you have taken the center and the bag is leaning on you. That is how close a bad guy will be in the midst of an assault. That is the range that all of your self-defense striking needs to work from.

Even worse, there are exceptions, but most threats will attack from flank or rear in an assault. Again, if you see it coming, if a guy squares off at the sparring distance you are used to, it is not self-defense. Not only must your targeting and power generation adapt to different ranges, but you need to know how to damage someone behind you.

Expect part of your body to be controlled. Both good guys and bad guys naturally index—grab the opponent to make hitting with the other fist more accurate. Some go further and have practiced immobilizing a body or yanking someone off balance simultaneously with a strike or stab.

All of this may happen in an enclosed place with bad footing and limited visibility.

Self-defense at Level 5 or above is a desperate situation. It won't be pretty. Everything you learned about timing in sparring flies out the window. You may have been shoved against a wall or vehicle, unbalanced, awkwardly twisted, or falling. You may be reeling from a punch or kick or you may have been stabbed or shot. But you still must be able to fight, and fight effectively, in cramped, close conditions while unbalanced, held, and possibly with your structure compromised, despite being injured, and with limited or no visibility.

Piece of cake.

Causing Damage

As mentioned previously, Level 5 is about damage. You are no longer trying to discourage or control bad behavior. You are trying to make the threat *incapable* of bad behavior. Level 5 is all about breaking a human being.

In truth, it rarely works that way. Humans, like all animals, are physically tough and can survive a tremendous amount of damage. Really dedicated individuals have continued to fight or save others while literally shot to pieces:

- Jacklyn "Jack" Lucas was just sixteen years old when he dove onto two Japanese grenades to save his squad mates, taking more than 250 pieces of shrapnel into his body. He was hit in every major organ, including six pieces in his brain and two in his heart. And he lived.
- Matt L. Urban was shot seven times, including once in the throat, yet managed to kill 116 German soldiers in one day during World War II. He survived to become the most decorated soldier in the history of the U.S. armed forces.
- Jacksonville police officer Jared Reston was ambushed and shot seven times with a .45 caliber semi-automatic pistol yet managed to turn the tables and kill his attacker. He was hit three times in the torso and once in the chin, elbow, left thigh, and right buttock, yet he survived.
- John Finn was hit 21 times by bomb and bullet fragments as he tried to hold off Japanese planes with a machinegun during the attack on Pearl Harbor. He refused to leave his post until he got a direct order to seek medical attention.

Humans take a lot of breaking. Usually.

Sometimes it goes the other way, and a little breaking raises the stakes, makes the predator re-evaluate his game plan. When a rabbit turns on a coyote and kicks it, and the coyote leaves (or a cat makes an alligator back down), it is not because the prey did so much damage the predator was impaired, it just raised the stakes beyond what the predator was willing to pay.

This may sound like we are talking out of both sides of our mouths. Sorry about that, but this isn't a black and white issue. Every encounter is different. Nevertheless, it is about damage, which will usually work because of discouragement. So you see, both of those things are true. Humans take a lot of breaking, but often that is enough. What is important is that, if you are justifiably at these survival levels, your focus must be on damage. Let the threat work out his own psychology. If he quits because he is discouraged and leaves, fine. Freaking fantastic! If not, you do not stop until you are safe.

Dealing damage at close quarters under surprise, the essence of Level 5 hinges on three principles: timing, power generation, and targeting. If you have studied a striking art, these are the same concepts that make any strike work. The difference in Level 5 is the context.

Timing

We are dispensing with this one first because it is both the easiest and the one where everything you know from sparring is wrong.

Timing in sparring is a cross between a chess match and a jazz jam session. It is a complex, highly developed art and skill. In the mix of complex distances (centerlines, of course, but also reach with different limbs and range to different targets), differential speeds (yours, his, leg and hand, and bob and weave speeds), and personalities, there is a balance of offense and defense, and psychological and physical skills that make timing one of the big equalizers. A small man with superb timing can often easily defeat a big, strong man with shitty timing.

That's all cool. And none of it applies.

Ambush changes everything. The distance and the facing (threat to your back or flank) are chosen by the aggressor. He will be right at the range where his strikes will create the most power. The critical distance line, or step, or half step to develop the range that you rely on in sparring was crossed before you knew what was happening.

Speed is based on several factors, but the flurry of attacks will probably spike your OODA loop (sometimes referred to as "Boyd's Law" for military strategist Colonel John R. Boyd who codified it as a way of quantifying reaction times in combat). OODA stands for Observe, Orient, Decide, and Act. In laymen's terms, it is a cognitive cycle you must pass through to figure out what the hell is going on, determine your preferred response, decide to take action, and counterstrike. Several microseconds may pass, although it could possibly take minutes if you are frozen. All of your legendary speed in the ring will be pissed away as you instinctively wait for your opening or the break in his timing that you would usually exploit.

Your concepts of offense and defense are out the window under an onslaught of damage. He is not defending himself, and is counting on the swift repetitive damage to keep you from counterattacking. That approach allows him to put everything into attacking you. To defend each of his attacks AND counterattack, you must be twice as fast as he is, likely twice as fast as a human can be.

And the personalities. Everyone has a fighting personality. If you have sparred, you have developed one. The ice-cold counter-striker. The guy who dominates the center and owns the ring. The tricky one... Yadda yadda yadda. Who cares? It takes time to access that mode. You know when you are going to spar, and you have time to prepare. Even assuming your normal fighting personality has any value under an assault (most don't), you won't be assaulted when you are in that mode (unless your attacker is a blithering idiot).

Whether the threat hit you with complete surprise while you are in your nine-to-five brain, or he distracted you with the interview, or he's a charm predator who used his social skills to put you in social mode, or the threat let the tension build up until you were adrenalized beyond what you could handle, you almost certainly cannot access your fighting personality. You don't get to pick what kind of mind you will have in an assault.

The threat's personality will be unlike anything you have experienced in training. This is not a partner dedicated to helping you get better. This is not someone that, under the doctrine of "mutual benefit and welfare," will work to NOT injure you. This is not someone who will respect a tap or a point.

Your predator may be a scared kid feeling like he is losing control on his first crime and does not know how to regain control without resorting to extreme violence. It may be a hardened felon who will use extreme force without any thought of you, just a quick assessment of the odds of getting caught. It may be someone who enjoys the feeling of domination as he makes someone bleed and beg. It is very, very unlikely that you have hit any of these personalities in normal training. Most instructors would not let a uncontrolled predator anywhere near their *dojo*.

That's all the reasons the timing you have learned will not help.

Here is what will. Timing in a real-life assault is simple: You are at Level 5. You need to put some damage and kinetic energy into the threat. You hit the threat when you can.

You see an opening? You hit it. That simple. You hit it fast and you hit it hard, and you keep hitting any opening that you see until you can safely escape.

Regardless of incoming damage. Regardless of whether it is a scoring target. Regardless of whether you can hit it with a proper technique.

Timing under assault is simple. You hit what you can when you can.

And keep hitting.

Until the threat is no longer a danger to you.

Power Generation under Adversity

> *"The unforgivable crime is soft hitting. Do not hit at all if it can be avoided; but never hit softly."*
>
> —Teddy Roosevelt

Once you have been doing it for a while, generating power when you are striking a heavy bag, *makiwara*, or BOB is not all that tough for most martial artists. But it doesn't work so well when you are losing. When your structure is compromised. When you're bleeding and in pain. That is when it's tough to hit hard. But that's when it is absolutely necessary. You will end the situation only by getting kinetic energy onto the threat in a place that will put him down.

The threat is not afraid of your strength or physicality. If he were, he would have attacked someone else. Either because you are smaller and weaker, or because you are already injured, or because he is able to position you in such a way that he is confident you cannot apply power, the other guy is not worried about you.

Most of what you know about power generation is based on foot placement and distance. That is good and if you hit hard with specific techniques at specific distances, you should be working to get at that distance, but the threat usually won't allow you to start there.

We are not going to concentrate on this kind of power. Usually the threat has already neutralized it. We are going to concentrate on the cheats that work up close and personal:

- Using a tool.
- Using the environment.
- Using torque.
- Using gravity.
- Using momentum.
- Using aggressive forward pressure.

Using a tool

You are not an ape. Use a tool. This is the thing that trained martial artists forget most often. It is so obvious that we are almost too embarrassed to write it: *use a tool.* There is a reason that no one in all of recorded history has voluntarily gone into battle unarmed; to do so is stupid.

You will not be in control. That's one of the hallmarks of high-level (5 and 6) survival fighting. The odds of your having a weapon in hand are close to zero. But if you can access a tool, use it.

You can hit harder with a slightly curved paperback book than with your hand. A pencil can do things your finger strikes cannot. Your computer bag or purse makes a fine flexible club or flail and there is no chance of breaking your own hand like with a fist blow to the head.

The challenge with tools is that they often raise the stakes to Level 6. Tools are weapons. You need to be able to justify them. The type of tool can be important too. In many jurisdictions, there are legal distinctions between deadly weapons and dangerous ones. A deadly weapon is generally defined as anything manifestly designed, made, or adapted for the purposes of inflicting death or serious physical injury.

The term includes objects like firearms, knives, swords, and explosive devices.

Use and carrying of deadly weapons, concealed or openly, is governed by state and federal laws. If you carry one, know the laws where you live and travel. Because of differences among the various states, a person who is lawfully permitted to possess a weapon in one state may be precluded from doing so in another. Generally, use of such devices during the commission of a crime enhances the nature of and penalty for that crime. For example, while striking someone with your fist might be considered simple assault (depending on the circumstances), doing the same thing with the butt of a pistol could become aggravated assault, a felony.

A dangerous weapon, on the other hand, is something that can be used to injure or kill a person, but was not expressly built for that purpose. Items like hot coffee, fire extinguishers, beer bottles, rocks, and vehicles (in some jurisdictions) can fall into that category.

One implication of this difference is that if you are carrying a deadly weapon, you may have a more difficult time claiming self-defense than if you happen to find a dangerous weapon lying around and use it in an impromptu manner. In the former case, you may have to prove that you were not looking for trouble when you left home carrying the device. The prosecutor will want to stack the jury with folks who do not carry concealed weapons and, depending on where you live, may be successful in doing so. Also, concealed carry permits are not available in all places.

On the other hand, a deadly weapon is typically holstered or carried in such a way that you can deploy it quickly and efficiently. When fighting for your life, impromptu weapons are not always available and suboptimal at best. There are trade-offs for everything.

We will talk more about weapons in Level 6.

Using the environment

Fights happen in places. Again, this is one of the truisms that is so obvious we feel stupid writing it. In most martial arts and martial sports, every effort has been made to keep the environment clean, uncluttered, and safe. Floors and even walls are often padded. The broken glass and, occasionally, used condoms and discarded syringes of some of the nastier places are noticeably absent. Grappling is almost never practiced with beer bottles or pieces of brick lying about conveniently.

Training without this stuff lying around is good for developing specific skills. But it also creates blind spots.

Real life:

> The gangbanger did something stupid, took a swing, probably. Side effect of years and encounters, I usually only remember the spectacular ones or the ones I learned something from. A simple takedown on a swing doesn't deserve memory space. What I remember is that he hit the ground face down, as I intended and then I noticed the baggy pants, sagging to knee-level. I stood on the crotch (not the threat's crotch, the crotch of the saggy pants). He was completely immobilized, pinned to the ground, both legs locked straight.

Training:

> The visiting aikido instructor slapped his hands to the inside of his knees as he knelt, causing his hakama to fan out in a beautiful vee on the floor. I thought it looked cool, so I imitated the action. My sensei shook his head. "We don't do that in this school." Dave told me later, "It looks pretty but you just step on the hakama and he can't stand up."

More damage at less risk to yourself is done when you slam a threat into a corner, more than anything you can do with your fist, foot, or elbow. Pushing a coffee table into his shin. The ground-and-pound on a concrete or asphalt surface: this isn't a match and this isn't an octagon. When the threat tries to take your face off, the slightest miss plants his fist in the unforgiving concrete.

Curbs and stairs are for tripping over. Doors are solid wooden lever arms when it comes to bashing and some doorknobs are set at a good height to chip the tailbone.

A parked car, park bench, or brick wall. They are all useful tools—if you smash the other guy into them. That's the cool part, you do not need to draw or reach for anything. Just be aware of your surroundings and use them strategically. Knocking someone into an object tends to play better in court than picking something up and hitting him with it anyway.

The environment can be your friend. Use it.

Using torque

Explosive rotation can add power to your blow. An easy example of this is an inside-chest block. Have a partner stick his arm out simulating a punch and strike it with the inside of your forearm by raising your arm and swinging straight across. Even if your arm is accelerating at the point of impact, this move should not hurt your partner's arm. If you simultaneously rotate your forearm as you connect the blow should feel much more powerful. Now, do it again, but explosively like a sneeze.

The same principle applies to a hammerfist or backfist strike. Even if you cannot move very far, rapid rotation at the moment of impact can magnify the blow. You can do this move with a standard punch too. For example, start with a standing fist and then rotate into a forefist punch. Be sure to keep your elbow down, body aligned properly, and accelerate as fast as possible. In this manner, you can hit fairly hard even with a very short range of movement.

Torque is useful when you are very close to or tangled up with your assailant. Explosive rotation adds power to what may otherwise be an ineffectual blow even when your structure is suboptimal or compromised.

Using gravity

Using body weight is one of the big equalizers, especially for small people and especially in close quarters where you may not have the room to put momentum into a fist.

Odds are if you grab a bigger person by the head, you cannot pull him down, but if you jump in the air and swing off his neck, he will be lucky if hitting the floor is the only injury he takes.

The drop step is one of the most effective and simple methods for generating a lot of power. It gets missed, sometimes, but the body mechanics are found in every striking system. It was best described in Jack Dempsey's long out-of-print book*, *Championship Fighting: Explosive Punching and Aggressive Defense.*

The drop step is, in essence, deliberately falling. It uses gravity as a speed and power multiplier. The cool thing is that gravity doesn't telegraph. There are no tells to falling.

The concept is simple. Stand with your feet shoulder width or a little more apart and suddenly lift one. You will immediately begin falling to that side. If you do it right, which you won't at first. This is because trained martial artists have been told since the first day to always stay on balance.

Now some schmoe is writing in a book that sometimes it is very useful to fall on purpose.

So you go with your years of training and subtly, subconsciously, shift your weight to your left foot before raising your right. So you do not fall right away, but slowly, like a teetering tree. Furthermore, the shift of weight to the other side is the telegraph that the technique should not have.

If your right foot snaps up with no attempt to control balance, you will move, falling faster than you could step.

Often saying the words does not help. A trick you can use is to snap your right foot to touch your left knee as quickly as you can. The effect you want is not a step, but like a leg that has suddenly been removed from a stool.

Your foot will get back to the ground in time to keep you from falling down.

The drop step, properly executed allows you to deliver considerable power in a tight space and even to the rear or flank. Once you get the timing right, you can use the same principle even if you are falling uncontrollably because the other guy knocked you off balance. Strike at the moment of impact, using your weight as a power multiplier.

* You can still find the complete text on web sites such as www.scribd.com.

Using momentum

You will be pushed, pulled, lifted, hit, and jerked in a fight. Your base is disrupted. That is one of the reasons why trained people find power severely weakened. If you aren't prepared for it and get psychologically overwhelmed, the chaos of a fight will freeze you.

Understand that this chaotic movement is the natural environment of a fight. It is just the way things are. If you are a fighter, you should be comfortable with someone trying to swing you into a wall or shove you down the stairs. This is normal. You may have to spend some energy getting used to normal.

Judo *tachi-waza randori* (standing free sparring) and *sumo* are both excellent ways to get used to the dynamic of moving and being moved.

When you become comfortable with being moved, this chaos and loss of base become gifts that you can use to make your application of force more effective. The threat grabbing you by the hair and forcing you down may also be forcing you into his own knees making it easier to throw him. The threat pushing you into a wall is also giving you force so that when you twist, he will plant hard.

Mentally, using momentum is easy. Rather than stop the threat's force, you keep it going, maybe with some slight steering so that he runs himself into a solid object. Or you throw your short punch so that the threat is moving into it, adding his power to yours. Or you simply get out of the way.

The dull bong from the booking counter sounded wrong. Unusual. Any unusual sound in a jail is likely to be bad, so I headed that way. One of my officers was standing over a big drunk who wasn't moving much.

"G, what did you do?"

"Nothing, sarge. I just stepped out of the way."

The drunk had tried a football rush on the officer. When the officer simply stepped out of the way, the drunk drove his own head into the stainless steel counter. The officer never touched him. The drunk needed an ambulance, nevertheless.

Using momentum can get complicated and it is something learned best by feel. If the threat is moving, he has momentum based on his weight and trajectory (speed and direction). If you can manipulate his trajectory, you can exploit his momentum.

Any time that you are moving, or being moved, you have momentum that can be used in a fight. Even being yanked off balance backward by the hair, one of the most common attacks on women, can be exploited by jumping or falling with the pull and leading with an elbow.

If the threat is hanging on to you and either or both of you are moving, you make a system with possible rotational momentum and a shared center of gravity. That is a fancy way of saying that if the threat swings you in a circle, spinning you around his center of gravity and you suddenly drop, his own force will cause him to swing around your center of gravity. His lifting you onto your toes adds power to your uppercut.

Pretty cool, huh?

Using aggressive forward pressure

Sparring, often, is a game of distance and timing. That means that there is a lot of circling and backing up. Those actions can become habits. Practitioners try to maintain their separation, just out of the critical distance, and that becomes their comfort zone. It is an assumed condition that people who spar a lot often center their tactics and strategy around. This approach works great in the ring. It helps them win the competition. Unfortunately, it's worse than useless in most brawls on the street.

When you are under attack and overwhelmed, the dynamics change considerably. We are aware of two reliable options that can help you turn the tables on your adversary. Neither are techniques, nor are they wholly mindsets. They are an aggregate of attitude and principles and strategy. In the first option, you turn fear into anger and with aggressive forward pressure, ignoring damage, and taking the offense completely. You fight your way through the threat to safety. Colloquially, that's going "ape-shit" on the other guy.

The other option is rare and we do not know anyone, no matter how solid their training, who has been able to access it the first time they were attacked. Or even the tenth time in many cases… But there is a place where you go icy calm and everything the threat does and is becomes merely a gift or tool to exploit. Train for this skill, but do not count on the mindset. Not the first time.

If all else fails, aggressive forward pressure can get you out of many precarious situations. You will need a certain level of structural integrity (spinal alignment, balance, etc.) and a lot of attitude in order to pull it off. It works quite well when you can make it happen, but it is not the end all, be all by any means. Nevertheless, aggressive forward pressure can be a good way of turning the tables on your attacker so that you have a decent chance of regaining control of the situation.

Targeting

There were only two combatants involved, but it took eight of us to break up the fight without hurting anyone, four officers, three security guards, and myself. Once we got the participants separated we began sorting out what happened.

The surly guy was cussing, spitting, and arguing vociferously, but his friend just stood there impassively. The quiet guy was huge, a good head-and-a-half taller than me, but he hadn't been directly involved in the fight and didn't appear to be a threat, particularly not with all the authorities around. I wasn't paying him much mind when I suddenly realized that his elbow was speeding toward my head. I didn't have sufficient warning to dodge or block, but I was able to roll with his blow, spin around, and land an uppercut to his side. Just as I felt his floating ribs snap, he seemed to teleport away. Two officers had grabbed him from behind and dragged him onto the ground.

In the confusion, no one realized that I'd busted his ribs, least of all him, at least until some fifteen or twenty minutes later when he was allowed to stand back up to be escorted out of the stadium. I could see him wincing in pain with each step. He took a full power shot to the side that didn't even slow him down during the altercation while I received but a glancing blow to the temple, yet I suffered headaches, nausea, blurred vision, and ringing in my ears for almost a week. It wasn't until the symptoms began to ebb that I belatedly realized that I'd had a concussion.

Y'all need a little introduction to medical damage.

Shock

Shock is the big daddy of medical damage. Many years ago Rory's EMT instructor told him that shock was the only thing a human can die from. Everything else, from motor vehicle accidents to gunshot wounds to cancer to old age were just different ways to get to shock.

So what is shock? The inadequate perfusion of tissue with blood and/or oxygen. If the brain does not get blood, the brain shuts down. If the brain does get blood, but the blood is not oxygenated, the brain shuts down.

This holds true for every other organ and tissue. You shut down organs or make an organism die by denying oxygen to critical tissue. Simple. Maybe too simple.

There are four basic kinds of shock. Hypovolemic shock means there are inadequate fluids in the blood stream for whatever reason (dehydration or hemorrhage). When someone bleeds out or starts going all shocky from a ruptured organ bleeding internally, it is hypovolemic shock.

When the heart is not pumping enough, that's cardiogenic shock. It does not come up much in fights.

Anoxic shock is when the blood is getting there, but it is depleted of oxygen. Suffocation and strangulation are not the only way this happens in a fight. Some people forget to breathe. Sometimes you can put your body weight on the threat's lower ribs and he will become weaker and weaker as he struggles against the pressure.

Neurogenic shock means the brain has failed at regulating the circulatory system, usually dilating the blood vessels faster than the heart can compensate (this is basically what happens when you stand up quickly and get a "head rush"). Sufficient damage to the brain, especially to the brainstem at the top of the spine, can mess up the circulatory system in a number of ways.

There is a special subcategory of neurogenic shock called psychogenic—nothing went wrong in the brain but following a psychological or emotional trigger, the person faints. This is what happens when someone with no stomach for a fight gets a Hollywood knockout after a light tap. It wasn't a knockout. The dude fainted.

This section is not meant to be a medical text. Here is the deal: you shut off blood or breath, the person stops. The brain shuts down. Sometimes it takes a while—over a minute to suffocate someone to unconsciousness. Sometimes it is relatively quick, as fast as seven seconds for a good carotid strangle, but seven seconds can seem like a long time in a fight.

To shut off the brain quickly is hard. The Hollywood knockout, where somebody gets hit in the head and wakes up fine a little later, is pretty much a myth. If someone passed out without neurological trauma, they did not get knocked out. They fainted.

People get immediately knocked out one of two ways: (1) the skull is hit so hard that it actually intrudes in and disrupts the brain or (2) the forces slap the head around so fast that the brain bounces off the inside of the skull. There's actually a third, more-or-less: sometimes, with enough torsion, the brain tears away from vessels and anchors, and the situation will get really bad.

I met a homeless guy, Danny, recently. Danny awoke one night while being beaten by another homeless guy with a hunk of rebar. The assault broke both his arms in numerous places, shattered his right hand, and staved-in part of his skull. Where his right temple should be is a 2 ½ inch long, nearly inch deep dent. When that wound was fresh it required 37 stitches. A year later, Danny is just fine (insomuch as a guy who chooses to be homeless can be anyway). He has no memory problems, speech impediment, migraines, or any other lasting effects from the assault, save for the dent in his head and some pretty wicked scarring. Describing the attack he said, "My destiny is to die on Indian land. Living here in White Center, I knew it wasn't my time."

Even this extreme trauma usually does not result in a loss of consciousness immediately. Many of those who lose consciousness pass out later as part of the brain swells like any other bruise. The brain gets squeezed.

Taking head blows even without ever getting knocked out can still cause "microconcussions" that have some very bad long-term effects. We think everyone should try boxing, at least until they get over the fear of being hit, but we do not recommend anyone stay with boxing for an extended period of time.

There are some possibilities for non-concussive unconsciousness or unconsciousness without significant brain trauma. A good example is strangulation (sleeper holds, vascular restraints...there are many euphemisms) where the person goes out for twenty seconds or so. Unless there is a pre-existing condition (e.g., heart problem, arterial plaque, or blood vessels weakened by excessive drug use), there are no ill-effects.

That is brain trauma. Other tissues can be torn or injured in different ways.

Organ Bruising and Injury

Most muscles, when hit, bruise. That is just swelling from small blood vessels being torn. The bruise can make the muscle tight and painful. Seriously, though, if you've never had a bruise why are you reading this book?

Significant intrusion into the body as well as really horrific levels of force can injure organs. Some organs, when bruised, bleed. Sometimes significantly. Other organs can be lacerated (cut) by shards of bone. The horrific levels of force mentioned above, like deceleration trauma when a vehicle hits a tree can actually tear organs. That does not come up often in a fight. Internal bleeding, especially with weapon trauma or falling, can damage certain organs like the liver and spleen.

Broken Bones

Bones can be broken. It is not easy. Long slender bones tend to be weaker than short, heavier bones. Narrow ribs and clavicles break easier than the thick femur or humerus. It is almost impossible to break a free-moving bone. In other words, if a hand is in the air, it will be very hard to break a forearm even with a club. Brace the hand against a hard surface and it becomes much easier.

Fracturing bones rarely causes someone to stop fighting. A guy with a broken bone can still pull a trigger. A man with his right arm dangling at his side can still use his left. But a fracture tends to make people not want to play anymore.

Joints and Sprains

Joints are generally more vulnerable than bone. A skilled twist or hyperextension can stretch ligaments and tendons beyond their design specifications. If they stretch far enough, the joint can be dislocated, which means the bones are separated from each other and do not go back into place. A sprain is when the bones are separated but do return to proper positioning on their own.

Sprains are injuries. They hurt and tend to swell, which makes it hard but rarely impossible to use that joint. Dislocations tend to be more painful and the limb is often nearly useless. Rory has made his arm under a dislocated shoulder work, but he has never made it work well.

The tendons and ligaments can merely stretch (sometimes painfully, rarely physically debilitating) or tear. Tears can be severe, often disabling the limb, or so minor that you may have dozens of small tears in various places right now and not know it.

Okay, that's medical damage. Not every type of injury by any means, but a sufficient introduction for understanding what might happen in a fight. Now, let's get legal for a second. If you inflict a serious physical injury on another person, there are repercussions. From NY State Penal Code Chapter 40 Section 10:

> *"Serious physical injury" means physical injury which creates a substantial risk of death, or which causes death or serious and protracted disfigurement, protracted impairment of health or protracted loss or impairment of the function of any bodily organ."*

There it is. You are intentionally trying to break someone. At Level 5, you are hoping for something that isn't permanent. This desire affects your choice of targets. Damage depends on how hard and accurately you strike as well as what you hit with. Most martial artists can deliver a pretty strong blow under optimal conditions using their fists or unshod feet, but a Level 5 situation often requires help from some sort of solid object. Threats who are stimulated by adrenaline, fear, drugs, alcohol, or even sheer willpower may not be incapacitated by anything that is not immediately physiologically disabling, even if mortally wounded.

If Level 5 isn't working, you might have to escalate to Level 6. Immediately.

One final thing to think about. A danger of Level 5 that most folks don't consider is exposure to blood-borne pathogens (such as hepatitis B, hepatitis C, or HIV/AIDS). Any time you break the other guy's skin, there is a potential risk. This risk is increased if your skin is broken as well, one of many reasons why punching a threat in the mouth is stupid.

In the next few sections we will cover specific targets that you may consider attacking to cause damage to a threat. Nothing's perfect, nothing is a panacea. The particulars of each individual encounter will vary, so the tactics you use must reflect the nature of the threats you face...

Foot

The foot is a useful target, particularly if your goal in a confrontation is to escape. Traditional *kobudo** systems, such as Matayoshi, target the foot with *bo* (staff), *kuwa* (hoe), and *sai***, among other weapons, because the ancient masters knew that it was a tough target to defend as well as a good way to end a fight. With a weapon or even a powerful stomp, the small bones in the foot can be crushed with a

* A Japanese or Okinawan martial art featuring a variety of weapons forms derived from common agricultural tools.

** A traditional *kobudo* weapon, the *sai*'s basic form is that of an unsharpened dagger with forward curving projections rather than a traditional cross-guard. It was popularized in movies, such as *The Mummy Returns, Mortal Kombat,* and *Elektra.*

downward blow, disabling an opponent's balance and reducing his ability to move, fight, or chase you. A blow to the upper surface of the instep can damage the plantar and peroneal nerves causing pain throughout the leg, hip, and abdomen thereby weakening the leg. Digging your toe into the top of the other guy's foot at the base of his toes can cause excruciating pain too. While this will not stop him, stepping hard might help move him into a position where something more debilitating can be delivered.

Simply stepping on the other guy's foot can ruin his balance, keep him from evading a follow-on strike, or otherwise mess up his plans, but at Level 5 you are really looking for damage not disruption. You will likely have limited opportunities so it's best to make each one count. If the threat's foot is on the ground, the easiest way to injure it is with a stomp. Striking with the heel generally works best, particularly when you are wearing boots. If you are tied up with an adversary, particularly in a clinch, it may be possible to strike his foot without him seeing it coming, but you will need to be careful not to lose your balance in the process (which in a clinch is not all that tough as contact with the adversary will usually keep you from falling).

It is hard to practice foot-stomping with a training partner because most padding is inadequate to avoid risking damage. Timing is a critical component of a successful attack to the foot, so a useful partner drill is called "toe tag." It is best to go barefoot because this not only increases your sensitivity but also helps preclude injury. Start slow and work up to speed slowly. Here is how the exercise works:

- Begin with lunge punches (striking arm and leading leg both forward on the same side), moving forward and back in a straight line. As one partner throws the punch, the other blocks, deflects, or uses whatever defense is appropriate for his art and attempts to step on the puncher's foot in the process.
- Once you get good at catching the training partner's foot with your own, move on to reverse punches (striking arm forward, opposite side leg forward) and repeat the drill.
- When you become skilled at working both types of punches, start moving at various angles until you can find the other guy's foot instinctively without looking.

If you can step on the foot, you can stomp on it too. It is useful to practice stomping powerfully. After all, what gets trained gets done, and you are looking to do damage. Place striking pads on the floor and practice teeing off on them. This is a great way to perfect your technique and can be a lot of fun too. Once you become good with static targets, you can have a partner slide the pads along the floor so that you have something moving to aim for too. As with the previous drill, go barefoot so you will not damage the equipment. It will help reinforce proper striking angles too.

Combining the timing you get from playing toe tag with the power you can achieve from working the striking pads will set you up for success if you need to use this application on the street.

Ankle

The ankle can oftentimes be easier to target than the foot. You can stomp on it, of course. A downward blow to the knee that misses can be redirected to strike the ankle fairly easily in many instances. You can also attack it with a front or back kick. Short jabs with your toe or heel, particularly if you are wearing boots, tend to work well. These blows are hard to see and even harder to block or evade. You can entangle the other guy's feet, using your stance and movement to target his ankle or knee. The crescent stepping you find in many traditional martial arts facilitates this type of attack.

If the other guy is into high kicks, you may be able scoop-block and capture his strike, then punch or torque his ankle to cause damage. Similarly, you can work the ankle when grappling too.

The ankle joint may be hyperextended, dislocated, or damaged by a solid blow, causing severe pain, disabling an opponent's balance, and reducing his ability to move, fight, or chase you. A strong blow to the inside of the lower leg at the base of the calf can cause temporary paralysis of the muscles there. And it hurts like hell.

If, in the heat of battle, the adversary lands on the ground, it may be appropriate to stomp on his ankle as you make your escape, assuring that he cannot chase you. This technique can even look accidental, not that we would necessarily recommend that. Regardless, you need to be prepared to articulate why you took the action you did if you strike a downed adversary. Stuff like that looks really bad to witnesses. You must have legitimate reasons why the other guy is still a threat.

It is difficult to practice assaulting the ankle safely with a training partner. For this application, we recommend slow work. Use movement, angles, and body alignment during sparring to position yourself to hit the ankle with your strike, but do everything in slow motion so that no one gets hurt.

It is important to restrain yourself in slow drills. If you maintain a constant speed relative to your partner, the results will be much more realistic than if you accelerate to land the blow. Practice stomps, entanglements, and also kick defenses so that you can attack the ankle with both your feet and hands. When you capture and torque the ankle, go *really* slow so that your training partner can roll out of the technique without becoming injured. Overtorquing the ankle almost always injures the knee, and knees tend to heal poorly.

Talk to each other afterward. What works, what does not, and why?

Knee

I was in the zone. It was like I knew what every competitor I faced was planning to do before he tried it. And I beat them all with ease. Undefeated in a double-elimination, I reached the semi-finals. And then the accident happened.

My left knee was bent as I took a lunge step. That puts something like ten times your body weight on the joint. At that instant, he struck the side of my knee. It wasn't a legal target, or what he was actually aiming for, yet the combination of my movement and his momentum meant that his blow connected in just the right place at exactly the wrong time. I had this weird rubbery feeling as my knee lurched sideways, seemingly independent from the rest of my body, and then snapped back into place.

It felt really weird, but it didn't hurt. Until I tried to take another step. And fell. And couldn't put any weight on my left leg after I got back up. I found out later that it was a medial meniscus cartilage tear. And stretched ligaments.

He was disqualified, but I was done. Not just for the day, but for four months including arthroscopic surgery and rehab.

When the knee is bent, as it generally is in combat, it is not particularly vulnerable from the front unless you are wearing a steel-toed boot or using an impact weapon. If you strike the knee from the back, you can cause it to collapse but are not likely to produce serious damage unless the kneecap lands on something hard and/or jagged. The side however, is another story. When hit from the proper angle, particularly when the threat's weight is on the leg struck, his knee can be hyperextended or dislocated to disrupt balance and effectively take an opponent out of a fight. Ligament and cartilage damage often take surgery to repair.

While striking an adversary's knee can cause crippling injury, it does not appear as offensive on film as a blow to the face which, even when minor, can cause extensive bleeding. It is a very useful application if your goal is to escape. If, for example, you block an attack using a closing technique while simultaneously shifting to the outside, you may be able to strike the other guy's knee and run away all in the same motion.

Again, this technique can be practiced with a partner. Go slowly. Look for body alignment and positioning. Find ways to post the other guy's weight (e.g., grabs, pulls) in conjunction with your strike. Work into being able to hit the other guy's knee from any in-range position without looking. Sudden, instinctive knee strikes can be game-changers in a fight.

Ribs

A blow to the ribs rarely ends a serious fight. An adrenalized person may not even notice. The floating ribs (eleventh and twelfth ribs) are only attached at one end making them more vulnerable than other ribs to breakage. This damage is extremely painful and can hinder a threat's breathing and movement, even his ability to punch or kick effectively too.

> I've broken ribs with a hook twice. Both times the guy was wearing armor and I was wearing gloves. The second time, my opponent was wearing soft body armor (a ballistic vest) and we were both wearing sixteen ounce gloves. He had about 20 pounds on me. I broke two of his ribs. The match was over. That was a right hook.
>
> The first time, the opponent was wearing entry armor (inch thick foam with a semi rigid cover) and I was wearing my entry gloves—fingerless leather with padded knuckles. Steve had at least forty pounds on me. He went down faster than any head shot I've ever delivered.
>
> If, ladies, you ever wonder what it's like to get kicked in the testicles, take a liver punch. And guys, if you ever wonder what it would be like to have an eight-pound testicle get stomped, take a liver punch.

The ribs can be vulnerable to hooks, uppercuts, and palm-up center punches, among other empty-hand techniques. Elbow strikes are very effective here; particularly, a reverse elbow to the lower ribs. You can strike them with your knee or foot too, but kicking above the waist can be dangerous because it is slower, less direct, and easier to block, redirect, or capture than strikes to the knees, ankles, or feet. If you are grappling on the ground, however, a knee strike can work well. You can do the same technique with your foot if you are up and he is down. That sort of thing plays poorly in court unless he is armed, in which case you would probably want to target something more vital than the ribs. Or just leave. Quickly.

Ribs are common sparring targets, particularly when wearing protective gear. Heavy bags and BOB can help you learn to generate power when attacking this area too.

A note about kicks: Lawrence is primarily a karateka. Rory is a jujutsu-trained infighter. They kick entirely differently. Many of the objections to kicks in real fights listed above simply do not apply. Remember that this is at Level 5, so you are losing. When losing, you are being pummeled, crowded, and both your balance and your structure are being jacked.

Most kicks from striking arts won't fail under assault because you cannot even get them started. The front, side, snap, and roundhouse kicks are extremely range dependent. Merely stepping into a kick completely neutralizes the technique. Getting any foot into play when your head is being knocked around or you are grabbed and shaken—let's just say you do not need to worry about the kick costing you your balance because the odds are good you will not have the balance or the base to start the kick in the first place.

Infighting and infighting kicks are different. If you know what you are doing when infighting, you can have one leg in the air because both of the threat's legs are part of your support. Some of the techniques, the booted toe-kick to the ankle and the knee-to-knee pops, are quick and vicious. They take no room and almost no time. There are even a couple of effective infighting kicks that work above the waist...

Kidneys

It was supposed to have been a flag football game between two fraternities, but tackles were becoming the norm as our competitive natures came to the forefront. I wasn't wearing any padding, nor was anyone else for that matter, but didn't mind getting hit. Hitting the other guys was fun. Until someone fell on me hard, driving his knee into my kidney. I don't know whether or not it was intentional, but it felt like I'd been stabbed in the back. Pain shot all the way up into my neck. It took me several seconds before I could stand up. Limping off the field, I watched the rest of the game from the sidelines. There was still blood in my urine the next morning...

Most people aim too high on kidney shots. Less than an inch of the kidney is exposed below the ribs from behind on a normal person. This area is frequently targeted with kicking techniques because they can be reached in this fashion from the front, side, or back, although punches work well too.

A blow to this region from a blunt instrument can cause internal bleeding or shock. Near the kidneys is the hypochondriac region.

Located between the seventh and eighth ribs, approximately one hand width below the solar plexus, a blow to the threat's right side can affect the liver whereas the left side can get at the stomach or spleen. If an implement is used, blows to any of these areas can have fatal consequences due to internal bleeding. Death occurs by hemorrhage, a slow process. If medical attention is reasonably forthcoming, a kick or punch to the kidneys will rarely prove fatal. These blows tend to be quite painful, however, so much so that if your strike is ineffective, or not effective enough, you must escalate to other targets in order to stop your adversary.

Clavicle

The clavicle is a really nice target because it is relatively easy to break. A busted clavicle will physiologically disable an adversary's ability to use his arm to attack you. And it hurts like hell too. Unfortunately the clavicle is not always easy to target in the heat of battle.

One method of accessing the clavicle is a diagonal strike, say with a ridge hand. A whipping downward palm-heel strike can also work well. Another is a straight-in punch. That, however, requires the target to be leaning forward, such as he might be if he overreaches or you pull him off balance. This strike is easy to execute and has good power even at close range. While the BOB can help you practice this technique, it is too static to truly get a feel for how hard it can be to access this area. Consequently, partner drills work best. You are working near the head/neck, so use caution not to hurt each other while practicing.

Solar plexus

One of the advantages of striking the solar plexus is that it is not an area that looks particularly dangerous to hit or that is necessarily well defended in many cases. After all, you are punching the other guy in the "chest." But this is deceptive.

Located just below the xiphoid process, a blow to this area can shock the diaphragm rendering the recipient temporarily incapable of breathing. The blow is not going to kill him, but while he is worried about drawing his next breath, you can beat feet to safety. A powerful blow in this area, particularly when delivered by a blunt instrument, could cause internal bleeding, unconsciousness, and even death (though it takes a long time to die from internal hemorrhaging). More often than not, all you're going to do is knock the wind out of the guy if you strike him in this area.

Contouring is important when attacking the solar plexus. A fist is unlikely work; the impact is spread too wide. A single knuckle, the point of your elbow, or the end of a tactical baton can be very effective. A back-handed slap tends to get the perfect reaction. The solar plexus can be a challenge to hit in the heat of battle. Practicing on a BOB can help you identify the target, but it is only static. Partner drills can work best. Clearly, you must go slowly and/or strike lightly when training.

Groin

The game had been over for an hour and a half or so. I was walking along a bike trail on campus, heading toward the lot where I'd parked my vehicle. Between the darkness and driving rain I couldn't see more than a dozen feet despite the intermittent streetlights alongside the trail, so I carried a flashlight in my hand.

I heard them long before I saw them, a young couple near the stairs that led up to the student union building. I don't know what they were arguing about, but it appeared they'd been going at it for a while. As I approached she snarled something I couldn't understand followed by, "Be a man!"

For a moment he looked stunned. Then he hauled off and punched her in the face, knocking her clean off her feet where she crashed to the ground on the muddy grass beside the stairs. A foot to the left and she would have smacked her head against the concrete. While she lay, he began to advance, ready to strike her again.

I'd seen more than enough. "Hey asshole," I shouted.

When he whipped around to see who was there, I snapped on

the light, giving him 240 lumens full in the face. He flinched back, raising his hands to shield his eyes. And I kicked him in the groin.

"Why don't you pick on someone your own size?"

For a few seconds, he just stood there; then he let out a gasp and crumpled to the ground. He was still curled in a fetal ball gasping like a fish out of water when I helped the girl up and walked her back to her dorm. Since I was wearing steel-toed boots at the time, I probably should have pulled my blow. Probably.

The groin can be an effective target. Blows to this region can elicit pain, nausea, or vomiting in male victims. A firm grab can potentially be incapacitating. Upward blows to the pelvic girdle of a female adversary can elicit similar results, although it takes a bit more force and accuracy. But the groin is one of the best protected areas of the male body, so it can take a bit of trickery to attack it successfully.

And, there is a three-and-a-half-seconds rule. It takes about that long for the blow, no matter how serious, to affect the threat. A lot can happen in a fight during that much time. Worse yet, kicking certain people in the nuts simply pisses them off. Damage from a groin strike tends to be more psychological than physiological.

You can attack the threat's groin with your hands, knees, or feet. You could use your teeth too, but opportunities for that are rare and rather unpalatable for most. If you use your hands, you will most likely need to use angles and misdirection. Straight in can be really tough. The three main hand techniques for attacking the groin include the finger whip, grab, and lawnmower pull:

- The finger whip, or flyswatter as it is affectionately called, is simply a matter of whipping your arm toward the groin while keeping your wrist relaxed. As soon as your arm connects, shoot your fingers forward like a whip so that it strikes the groin and retracts as quickly as possible. This is much more painful than it sounds. Rory has taken a number of groin shots, including one that lifted him over a foot in the air. Only once was it immediately incapacitating and that was from a finger flick. Lawrence has had similar experiences. Nevertheless, it is unlikely to cause any long-term damage.

- The grab, or five-on-two as it is sometimes called, starts the same way as the finger whip, but once you make contact, you grab a hold and hang on tight. Squeeze as hard as you can. This technique can really get an adversary's attention.
- The most effective hand technique is the lawnmower pull. From the grab, turn your wrist over like you are checking the time and rip up and back as you would do to start a lawnmower. You can cause significant damage this way, even tearing off a testicle if you do it right. (In 2007, Amanda Monti tore a testicle off her boyfriend, Geoffrey Jones, with her bare hands…and tried to eat it.) While this will not necessarily end a fight, it has a reasonably good chance of doing so.

Straight in kicks to the groin can be tough to pull off unless executed from a very close range or with the element of surprise. Knee strikes can work from a clinch, and heel or back kicks can work if a threat grabs you from behind, but your structure may be compromised with such techniques. If you try a front kick, you are more likely to be successful with an upward angle than you would be going straight in. You can connect with your toes or shin, preferably straight up between the legs.

You can practice groin strikes in a variety of different ways. An elongated BOB or heavy bag can work well, but those things tend to be too static. Playing "cup tag" with a training partner can help you understand how tough it is to hit/easy to protect this area. Make sure you are wearing adequate protection and strike lightly. Get used to the angles and misdirections that work as well as those that do not.

Jaw

It was my turn to watch the door. Everyone at the party had had left their keys on a pegboard, and I wasn't supposed to give them back unless the person was sober enough to drive. About midnight Ron staggered up to me and demanded his keys. He was hammered, so I told him no, something along the lines of, "You've got to sober up first, man."

Well, he wasn't having any of that. He lunged for the keys. I got there first, grabbed them off the board, and twisted away from him. I told him no again, but he kept coming. He was bigger than me, and a serious asshole when drunk, but I wasn't about to let him kill himself or someone else driving home. Unfortunately, the other guys just thought it was funny. They were no help. Until he grabbed me by the throat and tried choking me.

I drove my knee into his stomach. It wasn't much of a blow but it did force him back. As he lunged again, I pivoted and hit him in the base of the jaw as hard as I could. Much to my surprise he crumbled to the ground. It was the first time I'd ever knocked anyone out. And I didn't even hurt my hand.

Thankfully, the next morning he didn't remember who'd hit him.

Any blow to the head can prove fatal. It is a dangerous application to attempt, although some targets tend to be safer than others. A blow to the jaw, particularly at the hinge, can transmit shock into the brain. The more the other guy's head whips around, the better the chances of obtaining a knockout from such a blow. Depending on whether you hit the chin or the base of the jaw, other injuries can include broken teeth, whiplash, or a broken or dislocated jaw.

It is a really bad idea to try to kick someone in the jaw unless he is on the ground, attempting a wrestling-style takedown (even then, most kicking experts cannot time the targeting on a rush), or otherwise has his head below the level of your waist. Consequently, most times you will be using your hand. If you are going to target the jaw, do not strike the chin with a closed fist. You're as likely to break your hand as you are to shatter his jaw, although you might accomplish both at once. A palm-heel strike is much more effective. With good form you can, however, punch the side or base of the jaw with a closed fist, although a quick turn of the head and you may wind up striking somewhere other than you had planned.

Elbow strikes oftentimes work well. Properly leveraged, you can generate tremendous power with it while simultaneously risking little damage to yourself when you connect. You can hit with the forearm too.

One way to safely practice jaw strikes is with hand shields. Have a partner hold a pad at jaw height and keep it moving around while you strike it. Get feedback on how crisp the blows are. Perform this drill statically, and again with both people (as the pad) moving to simulate the dodging and weaving that sometimes takes place during a fight. (You'd be amazed by how many people just stand there and pummel each other, even though movement and positioning are important aspects of fighting.) For solo training, a BOB much better than a heavy bag, although either will do.

Nose

Two fans had gotten into it. While it started as a stand-up fight, it only remained that way for a few seconds until one guy shot in, grabbed the other guy's leg, and took him down. Then he crawled up onto his chest, pinned his victim in place with his legs, and started raining blows down onto him. This was some twenty years ago, long before MMA became popular, but not so different than you'd see in the ring today.

Of course he did it on cement and the other guy didn't fall right, so dude on the bottom was in serious trouble. As I rushed to intervene, the guy on top suddenly flew backward screaming, blood pouring out of his nose.

We grabbed him so he couldn't get back into the fight, but I had no idea what had happened. I searched for some sort of weapon, but couldn't spot anything. Seeing the confused look on my face, the guy who'd been on the bottom said, "I shoved my finger up his nose. It made him let go."

Novel approach, that. Only time I've ever seen it.

Lawrence has had his nose broken seven times. The long-term impact was bad enough that he eventually had to have it re-straightened during sinus surgery to correct breathing problems. But a busted nose never knocked him out of a fight. Rory had his broken twice too; it only pissed him off.

It is really tough to get a knockout from this area without using a blunt instrument to augment your blow, but smashing the mid face can cause a lot of pain and bleeding. This is not likely to stop a committed adversary, but it may cause an attacker to rethink his choice of victims. Shoving your finger up a guy's nose can work too, apparently. The challenge with this area is that it can expose you to blood-borne pathogens.

The intermaxillary suture is located just under the nose at the philtrum. The nerves are very close to the surface in this area such that even a light blow can cause pain and watery eyes in most people. This sensitive area can also be used for control techniques when leveraged from behind such as pushing in and up to manipulate the head/neck and control the spine.

Several techniques can be effective in targeting the nose. The most obvious is the punch, although that can sometimes be hard to land, particularly the straight in variety such as a boxer's jab. Even if the other guy does not block, it might be possible to slip the blow. Doing so can be as easy as tilting his head, although it often takes a bit more movement than that. In some situations, a hammerfist works better, particularly if used as a riposte in combination with a block or deflection technique. The hammerfist can come straight in, but a vertical blow that lands at the top of the nose and crushes in and downward from there can really rock the other guy's world. Elbow and reverse elbow strikes are great ways to target the nose as well.

While the philtrum is more often used for control techniques, such as pulling one combatant off of another, you can add a finishing move to bring it to a higher level if necessary. For example, driving your thumbs into the threat's eye sockets or stretching and violently twisting his neck would accomplish this result. That could be hard to justify depending on the circumstances though.

Once again, the BOB is a fantastic way to practice targeting the nose as well as slow work with a training partner.

Ears

The ear slap is one of my 'A' techniques, ever since a girl in junior high school wanted to prove a point and put me on my knees with a double-ear slap. Maybe twenty years later, we were running a new set of training armor through its paces, seeing how well we could move in it and what the armor could and could not protect us from. Craig was wearing the armor, being the bad guy. I casually slapped his ear to augment a takedown. He didn't get up for a while. When he did, he couldn't hear anything on his left side. Through one of the best helmets on training armor made, I'd ruptured his eardrum.

A concussive slap to the ears can cause pain, disorientation, and severe trauma to the eardrum, particularly if the hand is slightly cupped. You can also grab and twist or even bite the ear to cause pain, but it is less likely to be fight ending than the good old fashioned "pimp slap" upside the head.

Eyes

I purchased the wrong type of coffee, a ground drip blend rather than the whole-bean variety I normally buy. When I popped the top of the vacuum-sealed can, a blast of grit exploded into my face and left eye.

Now I'm a pretty tough guy, a black belt in karate who's been in more than my share of violent altercations. And I wore contacts for years before getting Lasik surgery so I'm somewhat used to having "foreign objects" in my eye. Yet I experienced a nearly overwhelming desire to fall onto the floor and scream like a little baby. I didn't, but I really, really wanted to. If you've ever gotten smoke, sand, or similar substances in your eyes, you have a good idea of what I mean.

I stumbled to the bathroom and then took the better part of five minutes, and most of a bottle of eye-drops, to rinse the sludge out of my eye. It was still red and sore some five hours later.

So, what does a face full of coffee grounds have to do with self-defense? It is very tough to fight effectively when you cannot see. That makes an assailant's eyes an important target in a legitimate self-defense scenario. Compared to all our other senses, eyesight is dominant in its impotence for most people. It's not only how we view the outside world, but also how we acquire targets and defend ourselves against assaults.

Here is how to attack the eyes most effectively:

The thumb can be used as a wedge to displace the eyeball from the eye socket. This technique is done by placing your thumb against the inside of the bridge of his nose and pushing into the corner of your adversary's eye socket. Typically, you will use your fingers as a guide alongside the other guy's face. It works much better if you can support his head with your other hand or block it against an immovable object such as a wall, the ground, or a parked car so that he cannot move his head back or twist away.

When shoved forcefully into the eye socket, your thumb works much like a wood-splitting wedge, displacing the eyeball. This ultimate result is not typically a full removal of the eye from the socket, which is very challenging, but rather a stretching of the optic nerve that attaches the back of the eye and shoots excruciating pain into the brain.

A thumb to the eye can cause blurred vision, disorientation, shock, and in some

Eye attacks could be considered Level 6 because of the potential for permanent injury. On the other hand, pepper spray or similar substances can be used to temporarily blind an assailant, which would be Level 4, because it is actually only pain compliance, or possibly Level 5 because it is a weapon. (These things are not always cleanly categorized.) Either way, assaulting the eyes is dangerous stuff. In a legitimate self-defense scenario, the attack can be life-saving, but where it is not warranted, it can lead to serious jail time.

Not only can you cause horrific injuries, but you also let the other guy know that he is in a very serious confrontation. If you attack his eyes and miss, you are going to piss him off in a primal way, becoming the target of a lot more anger and violence than you might expect. Anything goes from that point on.

Anybody who wears glasses can probably relate to this situation. Having your glasses knocked off by another person, even accidentally, pisses you off. It is personal, it is primal, and it is instantaneous. Even in an accident, it takes real effort to control the instinctive reaction. This reaction gives you a glimpse of the type of response you can elicit from another person when you attack his or her eyes.

So, while attacking the eyes can incapacitate an adversary, it can enrage him too. Consequently, you need to know how to do it right. And practice effectively. The best techniques use either your thumbs or fingers. Either way, attacks must be executed powerfully, with resolve, and often more than once. The chances of failure without these three points are high.

cases blindness, more than enough trauma to let you escape to safety in most cases. If you actually displace the eyeball, the disabling effect is even more severe.

Fingers work too. If you are a trained martial artist, you almost certainly know how to do an open-hand block (e.g., *hiki uke*). After initially intercepting the opponent's blow, you can bounce off his arm and thrust your fingers into his eye socket. You can also rake across the eyes. Either way, whenever your open hand crosses in front of the other guy's face, you have an opportunity to reach his eyes. Even if you do not make contact, such movements can be distracting, leaving the adversary open to a follow-on attack such as a low kick or a knee strike.

Attempting to jab your fingertips straight into an adversary's eye can be challenging. It is fast and effective, but it is easier to block than other techniques and will will damage your hand if done incorrectly, so advanced training is necessary. Horizontal raking across the eye, however, can be nearly as incapacitating and can be easier to execute on the street. A good way to do this is to thrust your palm against the attacker's cheekbone, which serves as an anchor and guide. Then sweep away from the attacker's nose toward his ear dragging your fingertips across his eye. This motion is relatively natural, like twisting the lid off a jar.

Raking the eyes can damage the cornea, the outer lens of the eye. Scratching the eye with your fingertips can cause excessive tearing, light sensitivity, pain, and disorientation. While scratching may not cause sufficient trauma to let you escape immediately, it is likely to set up a fight-ending follow-on strike.

You can also use implements. For Level 5, the main implement you might use would be tear gas, pepper spray, or similar substances that cause temporary incapacitation. These hurt the eyes, but generally do not cause long-term injuries. We will cover self-defense sprays in depth in the section "Pepper Sprays," so we will not go into detail here. Also know that a hot cup of coffee, fire extinguisher, or similar impromptu weapon could also be used against the eyes with a very good chance of success. In the right range, such implements are nearly impossible to block, even if you do not have the element of surprise. However, you may be pushing Level 6 if you use them.

While the eyes can be a lifesaving target in legitimate self-defense situation, it is psychologically challenging to place your thumb or finger into another person's eyes with the intent to do damage. It is also hard to practice these applications safely with a partner. However, there are a couple of ways to practice eye strikes effectively. As with any training regimen, oversight by a competent instructor is strongly encouraged for the safety of everyone involved.

The first option is to use a BOB. Begin slowly and gradually build speed and power, practicing the aforementioned thumb and finger strikes against the BOB until you can do them instinctively.

The second option is with a live training partner. This training can be dangerous if done improperly, so exercise extreme caution. Cut an orange in half, duct tape it to a set of safety goggles, and give them to your training partner (despite the goggles, your partner would be well advised to keep his/her eyes shut tight and have a towel handy to wipe away any juice that gets through). Practice striking the orange with the aforementioned thumb and finger strikes. Striking against a real human, even one wearing this type of getup, can be disconcerting in a way that using a target dummy is not. Even if you use a BOB, it is a good idea to try the "live" drill too.

The first time you feel the orange give way beneath your fingertips should prove enlightening. It is important that a training partner be wearing the fruit to better simulate a real person than can be done with an orange alone or taped to a target dummy. You may well find that you are incapable of striking another person's eyes, something that is best known before encountering a life-or-death confrontation on the street.

Pepper Spray

I've been sprayed with OC (Oleoresin Capsicum) a bunch of times. It was required to qualify at my agency and we had extra requirements for the tactical team. Our qualification for the team was to take a full-face blast, then move to a heavy bag and deliver a series of elbow strikes; cross the room to another heavy bag and deliver knee strikes; deploy an expandable baton, find the next bag, and whack on the bag. Then we had to re-holster the baton, draw our duty weapon, and prone out a suspect. Then holster the weapon, handcuff and search the suspect (and find the concealed weapon), get him to his feet and escort him through two locked doors, maintaining control of a threat while using keys.

That was just qualifications. That was also a large part of why our agency set OC at Level 4, not Level 5. It is pain compliance. OC hurts and it makes your eyes water and usually shut, and often makes big streams of snot pour out your nose. But not to everybody, not all the time and even when it works, you can still fight.

My personal experience with OC has been less positive than most officers because most of the time I only got called when the spray didn't work—so there is sampling error. The ones that worked I didn't usually get involved in. So I've seen one guy with so much orange foam on his face that I thought it was a food fight and someone was throwing carrots…and the guy didn't react at all.

Had to go into a cell (with the team, thankfully) after a guy with two shanks didn't react to five magnum canisters of OC, which, by the way, made him extra slippery.

Watched one scrape the pepper foam from his face and eat it, staring into my eyes…

Anything we talk about here is a tool. Nothing is an answer.

Pepper spray is designed to temporarily distract or disable an assailant by affecting the eyes and mucous membranes. Most sprays come in small (typically 2 to 7 ounce) aluminum or plastic containers, although they are also available as pens, *kubotan*, and other assorted disguises including jogging weights, cell phones, and pagers (yeah, for some reason they still make ones that look like pagers). These containers hold the irritant along with a propellant, and sometimes other additives that increase the solution's viscosity, so that it can be sprayed roughly five to fifteen feet. Depending on the container, you typically get 8 to 10 one-second bursts per bottle. There are foaming, fogging, narrow, and wide-spray varieties. There are several common types of irritants available, but Oleoresin Capsicum (OC) is usually the most effective.

OC is a derivative of cayenne pepper. It is a more efficient inflammatory agent than tear gas CN (chloracetophenone) or CS gas (ortho-chlorobenzalmalononitrile) and causes an intense burning sensation, temporary blindness, a feeling of restricted breathing, and disorientation in most people. Unless the threat is affected by Chronic Obstructive Pulmonary Disease, asthma, or a similar condition, this "respiratory distress" is psychological. CS and CN can actually impair the airway, hence often considered a higher level of force than OC. The effects can last from 15 to 60 minutes depending on the concentration and environment in which it is used (and decontamination process). It is generally effective on drunken and drug-affected individuals, and even on dogs.

If you plan to carry a self-defense spray, be sure to practice with it. Classes are available from several training institutions where you can not only find hands-on instruction, but also get sprayed with the substance so that you will understand how it works. Many manufacturers sell an inert substance that operates similarly so that you can become used to disabling the safety and discharging the spray without having

While generally effective, pepper spray does not work all the time and can even become detrimental to a person who uses it. Some people are not very susceptible to chemical irritants. Alcohol and drugs can further reduce a person's receptivity as can glasses or contact lenses. Further, the use of a defense spray may enrage an attacker if it does not stop him, increasing the severity of the attack.

If the spray does not stop your opponent, it may also affect you as you try to grapple with him. It is slippery and may make the fighting terrain more hazardous and/or make grappling techniques more difficult to perform successfully. It can be dangerous to the user to deploy self-defense sprays in tight spaces such as bedrooms or vehicles. Wind, rain, and environmental conditions may reduce a spray's range and effectiveness.

Even though self-defense sprays are generally considered defensive in nature, they are prohibited in certain jurisdictions. Be sure to check the law before carrying them. For example, in the UK where it is classed as an offensive weapon, the sale and possession of pepper spray is illegal. In Washington, DC, pepper spray must be registered with the police. Pepper spray is also prohibited on some forms of public transportation such as airlines.

to think about it too much. Such practice is invaluable should you ever need to deploy the spray in an adrenalized state.

Because they are not very expensive, it is useful to buy extra containers and spray a "live" stream a few times at a safe outdoor location. Do not attempt to do this if you have not already felt the effects of the spray in a safe training environment with readily available medical personnel first though. You will want to be able to aim at the face of a moving target and hit reliably for a couple of seconds for best effect.

If you have gotten any spray on yourself, do not drive for some time afterward, especially not with the windows rolled up. When you sweat or take a hot shower afterward, residue on your skin will reactivate. Take a cool shower and do not, especially for your first hot shower, let the water flow over your sensitive parts. Not kidding.

Tasers®

Tasers® are less-lethal projectile devices that are very popular with law enforcement and security personnel. These devices use compressed nitrogen to project two small probes up to 30 feet or so, at a speed of around 160 feet per second. While Tasers come with various (effective range) cartridges, the models with the longest ranges are only sold to law enforcement, military, and aviation security agencies. While civilian models have a maximum effective range of 15 feet, they can be discharged at nearly any distance less than that. The civilian version also cycles for six times longer, 30 seconds versus five.

The most popular civilian model, the C2, is only six inches long and lightweight. It comes with a built-in laser sighting system to increase accuracy. But it has only one shot.

All models work best at ranges where the probes have an opportunity to spread out a bit in flight. These probes are connected to the

Taser device by thin insulated wires. An electrical signal is transmitted through the wires to where the probes make contact with the body or clothing resulting in a near immediate loss of the victim's neuromuscular control and the ability to perform coordinated action for the duration of the impulse. While Taser devices are generally effective, they do not always stop a determined attacker (except for the Taser ®Shockwave™ area denial weapon. It's a bank of 12 Tasers that fire all at once. For other models, evidence suggests that determination matters far less than obesity when combating the effects of a Taser). They do, however, have a higher one-shot stop percentage than bullets.

According to FBI statistics, 95 percent of officer-involved shootings occur at less than 21 feet, with approximately 75 percent taking place at less than 10 feet and a little over half at closer than five feet. These distances mean that most dangers take place in Taser range. You can use a Taser as a contact weapon too, incidentally.

While there is little evidence of Tasers alone causing accidental death—forensic studies typically find other contributing factors such as heavy drug use or excited delirium—some states are beginning to pass laws controlling the use and ownership of stun guns and similar devices.

Level 5 Conclusion

There are additional targets we have omitted, such as the shin, which can be painfully effective when struck with force. The goal of Level 5 is to break the threat's willingness to continue to fight, so we focused on areas that give you the best chances for success. After all, if you cannot escape to safety or otherwise resolve the situation at Level 5, you will have to take it to the next level. Additionally, the longer the fight lasts the greater your chances of being injured. Applications at Level 5 must be ruthlessly applied to end the confrontation as quickly as possible.

You have probably also noticed that the boundary between Level 5 and 6 is not black and white. There are way too many shades of gray, thus reinforcing the importance of being able to articulate the threat you faced and why you did what you did to escape it.

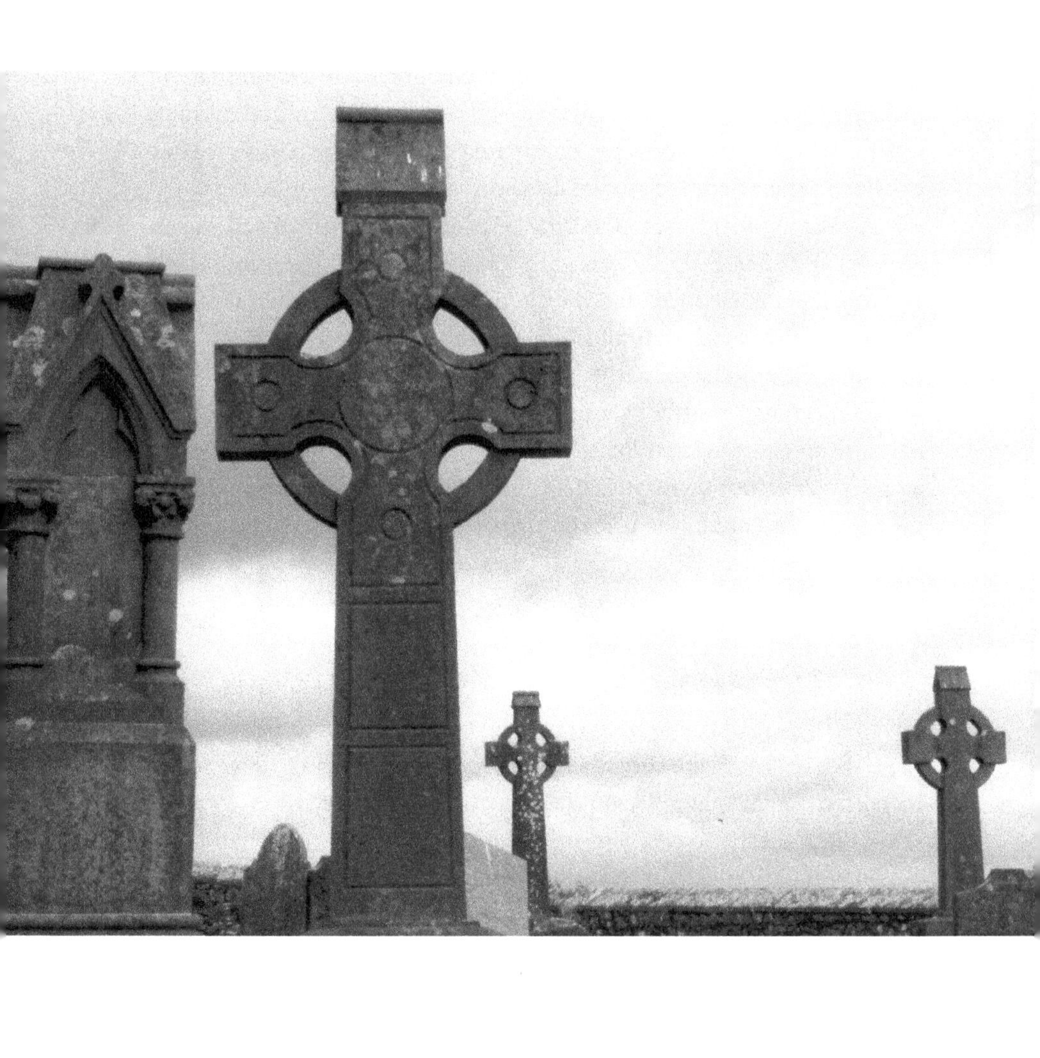

INTERLUDE—ON KILLING

"I don't shoot targets. I shoot men. Honestly, I figure I owe them that much.

"I know that when I kill someone I am doing to their family—their mothers and sisters and brothers—what the asshole who murdered my sister did to mine. My mother will never recover all her sanity from that. She won't ever stop grieving. Neither will I. Both of us are a bit broken. Making it by in a world that should still have her in it.

"Somewhere out there in this world there are families that felt that same split in their soul when they were told of what I have done to their loved ones.

"My sister lost everything to a selfish asshole who couldn't commit suicide without company. She would be 23 now. Would have graduated college. Maybe found a man. Maybe not. Maybe started grad school. Everything she ever would have done and been was taken from all of us.

"I do that to people. Some evil, some lost or misguided, some just doing what they can do to get some money. I don't feel bad about it. It has to be done. At the end of the day they set themselves in front of my rifle. But I figure the least I can do for them, and their families, is to acknowledge their humanity."

—Non-Commissioned Officer, U.S. Army,
Airborne Infantry.

Level 6 is about killing people. It is about deliberately taking a human being, an absolutely unique combination of genetics and history, and utterly destroying it. Someone who smiled at his newborn nephew. Someone who, from birth, was his mother's delight. There will never be this person again. Whatever he could have been is no more. Void. Empty. Nothing.

This is the manufacture of corpses and cripples. It is also the creation of widows, orphans, and grieving mothers. Your actions will create people who will never forget and never forgive what you have done.

The decision that underlies every decision to use lethal force is this: Whose mother will grieve? His or mine? Whose children will go to their beds tonight crying as newly created orphans? His or mine?

Everything up to this point can be a game. You can bluff in poker without saying a word. Debate is the verbal form of sparring. Touch can form the basis of seduction—and seduction, for right or wrong, can be played as a game. Submission wrestling and judo are competitions at Level 4. Boxing and mixed martial arts are the game version of Level 5.

You can argue that fencing and paintball are fun simulations of deadly force. Maybe. Except without the fear or the pain or the smell. No, we have not used killing people as a game since the gladiators… and even then most did not play.

There are no do-overs in deadly force. A bullet is one of those things that, once fired, you can never take back. If it is a mistake, it can never be undone. If you think of another option months or years later, you will have to live with the grave you need not have filled.

Never lose track of this. Some of you practice techniques in your martial arts that are readily capable of taking a life or crippling someone. Never forget what that means. Always treat it with absolute respect.

The application of deadly force can never be a game.

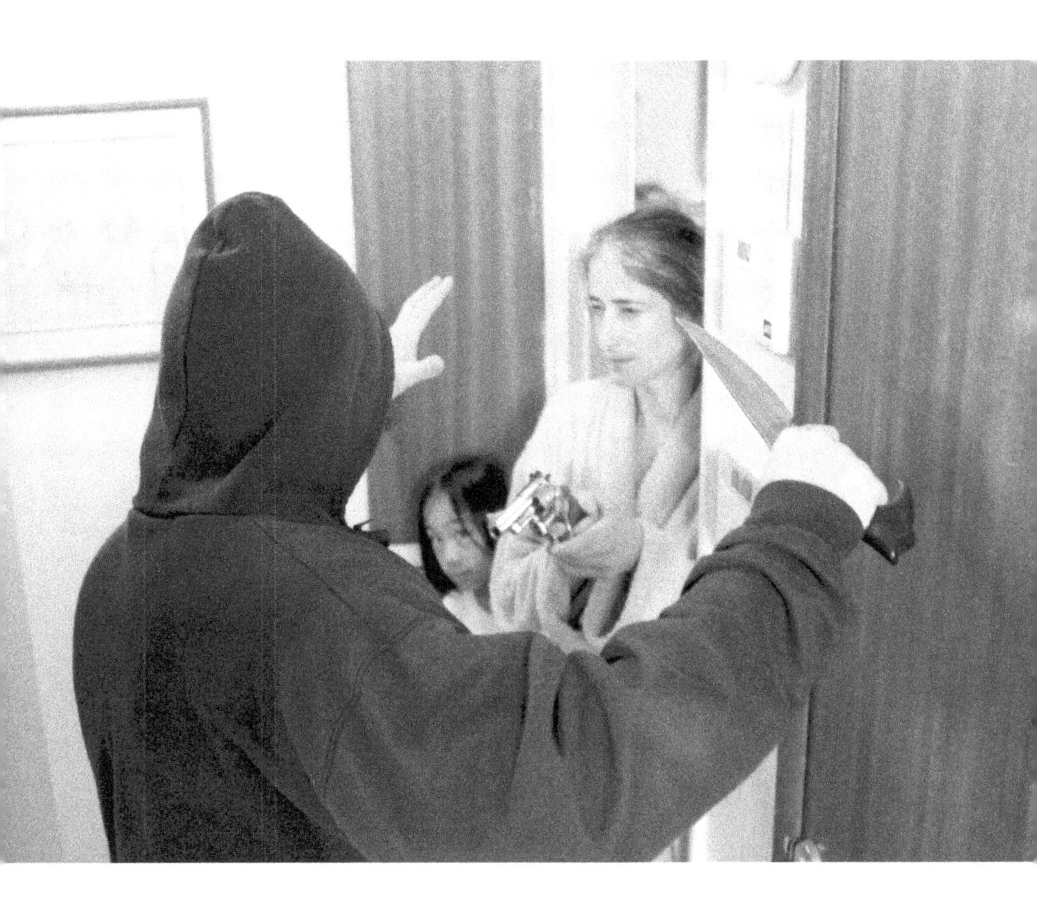

LEVEL 6—LETHAL FORCE

Gary Fadden was a salesman for firearms manufacturer Heckler & Koch. On February 24, 1984, he and his fiancé were driving their Ford pickup along Route 50 in Virginia. This was before cell phones became ubiquitous and he had no communication device inside his vehicle. But he had a competitor's rifle, a Ruger AC556 (the selective-fire, or colloquially "fully automatic" version of the .223 caliber Mini-14 carbine) that he planned to test as part of his job, in his truck that day.

While driving, Gary was cut off by two guys on a motorcycle and had to slam on the brakes to avoid an accident. Shortly thereafter he noticed a Chevy pickup with three passengers—two men and a woman—following closely behind him. Strangely, one of the male occupants suddenly began gesturing for him to pull over. Since he didn't recognize the folks in the Chevy, he ignored them. Until he suddenly realized that the passenger was waving a knife. And the driver had a gun.

He turned to his fiancé, saying, "We've got a bit of a problem here." Bit of an understatement, that, as things turned out.

As they entered Middleburg, a small town of perhaps 800, and came to a stop at a red light, the two men exited their truck and ran toward Gary's vehicle. One guy's hand was on Gary's door handle when he decided to run the light to escape. Unfortunately, the other guys jumped back into their Chevy and gave chase. Gary quickly accelerated to 95 miles an hour, but his vehicle's speed governor kicked in, keeping him from going any faster, so he was unable to elude the pursuing vehicle.

Unable to call for help, Gary desperately looked for a policeman he could flag down but didn't spot any patrol cars in the area. The chase continued for 22 miles, until they began to approach Chantilly Road and the H & K factory where Gary worked. Recognizing the location, he quickly planned to use his pass card to get through the plant's security gate where he could get into a building and find a phone to call for help. Unfortunately, the automatic gate mechanism took too long to open, so the pursuers caught up. One of them began to exit his vehicle before Gary could get through the gate. The nearest building was too far away.

Grabbing the Ruger, Gary told his fiancé to get down on the floor of the Ford. He threw open the door and stepped out where he was confronted by one of his enraged pursuers. The guy was average size, wearing ratty clothes, with stringy hair and a long beard.

"Stop or I'll shoot," Gary yelled.

Gary had never fired the Ruger. He knew how to disengage the safety, but was not sure which position the fire-control lever was set to, semi-automatic, three-shot burst, or fully automatic. He pointed the muzzle upward and fired a warning shot only to discover that the rifle was set on full auto. It ripped off nine shots before he could get his finger back off the trigger. Shockingly, this had no effect whatsoever. The bad guy kept closing. Fast. And he was carrying knives in both hands.

"Fuck you and your high powered rifle," he yelled. "I'm gonna kill you motherfucker!"

This time Gary aimed at the bad guy, firing six shots with one pull of the trigger. His assailant fell to the ground dead. Then the other guy tried to run him over. Moving quickly, got behind a brick planter to escape the onrushing Chevy. The pickup skidded to a stop and the driver bailed out.

"Fuck you! You killed one of the brothers! You shot him, you motherfucker," the guy screamed.

Gary's was prepared to fire again, but instead of using his revolver, the other guy looked like he was trying to hide it in his truck. Suddenly Gary realized why. The police had arrived.

But the incident wasn't over. Not by a long shot.

As it turned out, the Chevy driver was an outlaw biker who went by the name "Papa Zoot." He was unarmed when the cops arrived, but officers found two pistols in his truck, a .22 semi-automatic and a .357 Magnum revolver. The revolver had three live rounds and three empty cartridges in the cylinder. More spent brass was on the floor of the pickup, and a bag full of ammunition was open on the seat. Although no bullets struck his vehicle and he hadn't heard any shots, Gary was certain that the bad guys had been shooting at him during the chase.

The dead guy's name was Billy "Too Loose" Hamilton, another biker. Two knives were found on his corpse. Toxicology results from his autopsy showed that he had a .19 blood alcohol level when he died. He was hit by all six rounds that Gary fired, but he flinched away from the gunfire such that one bullet struck him behind the lateral midline, taking out a chunk of his spine.

You'd think that Gary had a pretty strong case for self-defense, right?

- Intent? Yup.
- Means? Absolutely.
- Opportunity? You betcha.
- Preclusion? Hell yes.

But, Gary was arrested that night. The charge? First-degree murder.

His family raised $60,000 bail.

He was vilified by the prosecution for "shooting Hamilton in the back." The press picked up not only on this point, but also on the fact that he'd used a fully automatic weapon.

The politics surrounding his case were ugly enough, but Gary soon discovered that Papa Zoot had purchased a .30-06 rifle and sworn a "blood oath" to kill him and his family.

At his trial, the prosecution brought Gary's attackers in to testify against him. They claimed that he'd tried to run over their biker brother, the guy on the motorcycle who cut him off earlier that fateful day, and that they'd chased him 22 miles trying to get his license plate number. They said that he'd tried to kill them, not the other way around. (Gary had all the proper permits; it was perfectly legal for him to possess the rifle.) The prosecutor made such a show of waving the machinegun around that the judge had to go out of his way to instruct the jury that the weapon used had nothing whatsoever to do with whether or not the shooting was self-defense.

When the jury found Gary not guilty on all counts, the prosecutor shouted, "You've let a murderer loose!" in open court. In front of Gary's mother.

> While Gary was ultimately exonerated, the bill for his legal defense was more than $45,000 (equivalent to over $100,000 today). It was eight years before he was able to pay everything back.

Level 6 is extraordinarily serious. If you are at this level, odds are good that someone is going to die. It could be you. And whoever lives, be it you or your adversary, is almost certainly going to jail. If convicted, that person will be doing hard time in prison.

Any blow delivered powerfully and deliberately to a vital area of the body could be construed as deadly force so long as it can be shown that it was struck with the intention, or predictable likelihood, of killing or maiming the other guy. Expect to be prosecuted for it. In Washington State, the definition of deadly force is "The intentional application of force through the use of firearms or any other means reasonably likely to cause death or serious physical injury."* Sounds a lot like Level 6 huh? This means that you are committing a felony. At a minimum, it is aggravated assault. More likely it's murder…

We have beaten you over the head with this detail already, but it bears repeating. **Self-defense is an affirmative defense.** You are admitting to the elements of a crime but offering an acceptable legal excuse for doing so because the threat had the intent, means, and opportunity to kill or grievously injure you or a third party, and preclusion was out of the question at the time. Further, you did not contribute in any way to the situation you found yourself in. A cornerstone of legitimate claims of self-defense is the innocence of the claimant. If you allowed a situation to escalate when you could have walked away (à la monkey dance), you're screwed even if the other guy pulled a knife or a gun before you took him out.**

It is vital to understand that Level 6 encounters carry supreme risk. Even bringing a weapon into play will not automatically stop a determined aggressor. Remember Jack Lucas, Matt Urban, and John

* Revised Code of Washington, RCW 9A.16.010.

** This is a bit of a grey area. California jury instructions, for instance, have a specific allowance for a fistfight where one of the fighters tries to raise the stakes to deadly force. It can still be self-defense. But not always.

Finn? It is exceedingly rare for a shooting victim to be stopped dead in his tracks by a single shot, even one to the head.

They had a saying in the Old West, "dead man's ten." It was a common experience for a gunfighter or knife fighter to continue the battle for another ten seconds after suffering a fatal wound. That was then; what about now? Have modern weapons changed anything? Not really. Loren Christensen wrote,

> *"I've had to fight guys even after they have been shot and they still fought like maniacs. I know of two occasions where suspects had been shot in their hearts and they fought the officers for several seconds before they crumpled dead to the ground... I saw two cases of people shot in the head—one person took five rounds—and they were still running around screaming and putting up a fuss."*

Mutual slayings are not all that uncommon at this level.

A defensive handgun instructor whose class Lawrence took reinforced this point, stating that it takes a fatally wounded person between 10 and 120 seconds to drop. You must expect a determined attacker to continue his assault even after he has been shot. Lawrence was taught to fire and move rather than stand in place as you might do on a gun range, staying vigilant until the threat was disabled and clearly unable to continue the fight.

It is even worse if you are unarmed. Justification for Level 6 includes an armed assailant or disparity of force. That means that if you're operating here, you're outgunned or outnumbered. Or both. With a weapon you may have a sporting chance. Without one, well it can be a roll of the dice...

This is Level 6 folks. And it sucks.

Mindset

One of the hardest concepts about explaining deadly force is that so few people have a frame of reference. They cannot really grasp what it is to use deadly force or what it will be like to exist even for a few seconds in the conditions that would justify it.

You can justify Level 6 when you think you are about to die. Take all the overwhelming loss and damage that justifies Level 5 (and makes it so hard to pull off) and raise it by an order of magnitude.

To put it another way—**if it makes sense to use Level 6, it also makes sense to hang onto your attacker, jump out a third story window, and hope for the best.** The essence of Level 6 is that you are going to die if you don't act. Given that baseline, that you are only a second from your own death, you have nothing to lose.

Perhaps the best you can hope for is to take the other guy out with you. Or to at least do enough damage and leave enough forensic evidence behind that the odds will be good that he will be convicted for killing you. Maybe, just maybe, you can do something totally nutso, take a long shot, and survive. You can do some pretty crazy things that have really bad odds, because you have nothing to lose.

Not a pleasant thought is it?

It is hard to truly comprehend this stuff. Tough to achieve a Level 6 mindset. To get your head into that place that gives you the will to win, or at least not lose, when your life is on the line.

In some ways, being skilled at competition actually makes it even harder. The reason for this difficulty is that the more intense the competition you have become accustomed to, the more ingrained your habits become. Sure, the experienced MMA fighter could gouge out an adversary's eye. Or crush his throat. Or break any other competitive rule in order to survive an assault. But thinking outside the box is extraordinarily tough when you're afraid, adrenalized, and fighting for your life.

Here is an example: If someone has you in a chokehold from which you cannot quickly escape, you are in deep yogurt. Once rendered unconscious, your fate is entirely in the other guy's hands. If he does not let off quickly, you are going to become brain damaged. Or die. One strategy you could attempt in a situation like this is to tap him three or four times, wait until he hesitates (or actually releases the hold), and then hit him with everything you've got. Lawrence has done this twice (in separate encounters) and it worked like a charm both times. The reason it is so effective is that grapplers are conditioned to stop fighting when their opponent taps out, signifying defeat. Don't expect to be able to pull it off more than once on the same person. It only works because it is a pretty much a one-trick pony. Your counterstrike had better work... It is a reflex action.

Deep-seated habits do not mean that folks who train for competition cannot succeed in self-defense, merely that it can be tougher for them because they have conditioned reflexes to overcome. If that's you, you need to instantly shift from competitive mode to combat mode. And that ain't easy.

Scenario training can help. The goal of such exercises should be not only to help you shift into combat mode, but also to help you find your limits because most fights end psychologically rather than physiologically.

You can, and probably should, attend seminars and professionally developed courses to gain experience, particularly where you can safely use weapon-simulators like Simunition™ and Shocknife® tools, or less-lethal devices like Tasers and pepper spray in relatively realistic conditions. These implements do not truly replicate the chaos and fear of real encounters, but they are a hell of a lot closer than rubber knives, paintball guns, or paper targets ever could be. Working with "woofers" who simulate bad guys, trainers in "bulletman" suits who can take full contact hits without breaking (usually) and the like is excellent.

"Will drills" that test your limits and help you learn to fight to the goal are important as well. Here are a few additional drills to consider:

Free-for-all drill

If you train long enough, *dojo* etiquette becomes ingrained. One of the challenges that experienced martial artists tend to encounter is working outside the box. Drills are, after all, "just" drills, so practitioners follow the rules even though they sometimes miss the larger picture.

Why are you doing the drill? What does "success" look like? If it is a competitive thing, success will be very different than if it's a combat simulation, which is not the same thing as a self-defense scenario. For example, if it is supposed to be light contact sparring, but the other guy is a foot taller and a hundred pounds heavier than you are, you don't run over to the weapons rack and pull out a sword to even the odds. Sparring is competitive, even when weight classes are not used. Success is not winning at any cost; it's scoring a point. If a training partner comes at you with a rubber knife and you are supposed to attempt a disarm, you do your best to make it happen, right? But if it's a self-defense scenario, then yelling for help while getting the hell out of there is more than likely the best approach. Why go hands-on against a dangerous weapon if you do not need to? In real life that's a losing proposition.

A simulated free-for-all brawl can be a really good way to learn the improvisation and develop the mindset necessary for street survival. The simulated brawl can be dangerous and takes a lot of preplanning, but it is worth it.

The "brawl" is generally done as a one-step drill for safety. That means that each participant gets one movement before the other guy gets a turn. This sounds sorta ho-hum, but with skill, the one step becomes extremely fast (though it really does not matter as long as everyone goes at the same speed and can be safe). Use a cluttered room. Nightclubs are preferable; you can often rent them for the day as long as you've finished and cleaned-up before customers arrive at night, but bars and warehouses can work too.

The game is played with everyone against everyone, using the environment. Everything is in play. Shoving people into corners, furniture, doorknobs, and other participants is fair game, expected even. Temporary alliances and anything else the fertile imaginations of the group can come up with is allowed.

Full weapons and "frisk fighting" rules are in effect, so you can use just about anything in the room or on the other guy to fight with. That means that street clothes are required, and firearms, knives, and other lethal implements cannot be brought into the facility. A common strategy is to pull implements off the other guy's belt, or out of his pocket, and use them against him. Unless you have experienced trainers in the space with thorough safety protocols in effect, do not do this drill. Everyone in the training area, including observers, instructors, and safety officers must be thoroughly pat-searched each time they enter the training area. No exceptions. If your safety protocols are lax or the participants let their egos get out of control, people will get hurt.

Instead of pool cues, beer bottles, and other impromptu weapons that could cause serious injury even at one-step speeds, simulations can be created. Rubber knives and plastic training guns you can buy, but you can make most anything else out of schedule-40 PVC*, foam pipe insulation, and duct tape. The PVC pipe is cut to length, shaped with a heat gun, and glued where necessary. Wrap with foam to create cushioned striking surfaces and seal with the tape to hold it together. That is a recipe for a rocking good time.

With his Tactical Team, Rory used to do this in extremely low-light conditions to add another twist. Once you get going, it's amazing how creative you can be with this drill. And what you will learn from it.

Find your limits

> The first time I tried riding a chairlift, I fell off. It wasn't far, perhaps a dozen feet, and I landed in soft powdered snow so I wasn't hurt. But it exacerbated my innate fear of heights. The acrophobia seemed to be getting worse over time, so I decided to do something about it. In high school, I took a summer job cleaning gutters. Since I had given my word to the owner of the company, and wasn't about to break that trust, I had to show up and face my fears every day for three months. It wasn't easy, but it was educational. Since then I've done a ropes course and even rappelled off a 75-foot tower. I still don't like heights, but I know that I can face them.

It is hard to know what you are truly capable of. Regular folks sometimes climb mountains to conquer their fears. Others participate

* PVC, or Poly Vinyl Chloride is used in commercial and residential plumbing systems. It comes in various thicknesses (e.g., schedule 40, 80, 120). The thickness is important when building training tools. Schedule 40 has the best balance of thickness and resiliency to flex under force without shattering in a way that can injure participants.

in Outward Bound or similar outdoor adventure programs that test their limits. Martial artists participate in thirty-man *kumite* and the like. Overcoming extreme challenges can be illuminating. It can empower you, or it can break you. There is a danger in such situations. But, it is useful to know what you are capable of, particularly when it comes to a struggle for survival. At Level 6, you cannot give up.

There are a ton of scenario training drills that can help. Here is one we somewhat hesitate to offer. It's risky. Odds are good that you will be a different person after you have completed it. Nevertheless, it is worth considering.

Find three to five experienced martial artists whom you trust completely. These guys need to have good skills and great control because this drill is going to be full contact. Use minimal protective gear—gloves, mouth guards, and hard-cups. It is a good idea to have trained medical personnel standing by just in case...

Your job is to spar against all of them at once. There are no rounds, no breaks, and no time limits. The only rule is that you are trying to hurt each other, not inflict lasting injuries. It's Level 4 and 5 work. Unless you manage to knock out all of your opponents, the drill continues until you are exhausted, physically unable to defend yourself. Then your opponents beat you for one full minute.

Going into a drill knowing that you cannot win takes guts. You will learn something about yourself by undergoing it.

Slaughtering an animal

Here is the deal: If you train in the martial arts and your technique fails, you will understandably be upset. Particularly if you have trained for years, decades. Often enough, when techniques work, folks become equally upset. Maybe even more so, because they are unprepared for results. The sound of breaking bones. The vision of a big man trying weakly to scream. You have been learning some nasty stuff and may be in for a surprise when you find out just how nasty it can be.

One of the biggest disconnects in martial arts training is that it is so easy to forget what you are training to do. An elegant throw used in the ring on a fellow practitioner who knows how to fall scores you a point. Wins you the match. The same throw on the street, performed on an average person who does not know a breakfall from a bowling ball, is slamming the other guy's head into the ground with enough force to shatter his shoulder. Or break his neck. A powerful, focused punch lands with enough force to concuss the brain or break or dislocate the adversary's jaw.

This is not mindfulness. To practice and to either forget or ignore what you are practicing is something close to unforgivable.

We had to put down Gazelle, a paralyzed goat. Put down means "kill." Maybe it means, "kill for its own good, for the cessation of pain." I went out early in the morning and dug the grave. It is a sin in my family to waste meat, but since the paralysis was probably due to loss of circulation the meat may not have been safe. I dug the grave close because I know that limp bodies are much harder to move than stiff ones. I took aim from about a foot and a half away with a .40 caliber semi-automatic handgun and pulled the trigger.

The shot was very loud in the morning quiet. I'd aimed for the sniper spot, the brainstem. We are taught that in a hostage situation, a direct hit on the brainstem will make the threat go limp, so they will not reflexively clench their hands and pull a trigger. I missed. I'm a good shot with a handgun. That means that on my best days, I'm about half as good as a TV hero. The miss (live targets move or I may have rushed the shot out of fear that Gazelle would move) was about an inch from my aim point, missing the brainstem but entering the brain cavity. It was a special expanding bullet and didn't exit the skull. Gazelle started shuddering and twitching.

She was dead—CSF (cerebral spinal fluid) and blood had erupted from both ears and her nose at the shot. Her eyes were fixed. I touched her eyeball and there was no blink reflex. She was dead, dead, dead. But the brainstem is old and animal, and it kept her legs jerking and her heart beating and her breath going in little raspy gasps. For about a minute. I think I watched that long because I was convincing myself that she was dead and I didn't screw up. But my wife was there (my excuse?) and it was hard on her to watch (oh, no, couldn't be hard on me... I've been butchering animals since I was a kid! Bullshit. It's still hard. I just do it more efficiently and with more respect and with clearer reasons now). So I fired again, this time hitting the sniper spot, and Gazelle went limp instantly.

People don't die much differently.

Can you take a life? Really? What's it like to have done so?

A friend of ours, Jack (Lt. Col. John R. Finch), relates,

"I have seen convicted murderers suddenly awake screaming from a sound sleep and try to run from what they later, I believe, honestly describe as the hands of their victims reaching for them through the walls of their room. As we staff intercepted these scared criminal patients, we realized that despite their crimes, there was more to their punishment than that meted out by the legal system."

Will you freeze and let yourself be slaughtered? Will you succeed only to wake up every night screaming in terror? Will you suffer from Post-Traumatic Stress Disorder (PTSD)? Or will you do what you have to, make the most of it, and move on?

Hopefully you will never have to find out. If you want to get a glimpse of what it is like, a mere inkling, in a legal and ethical way, try slaughtering and butchering an animal.

Yeah, really.

Hunting is okay, but it is really not an adequate illustration of what you need to feel. With bow or rifle, the distance is too great, the connection is missing. The skill going into the stalk becomes the focus, not the death, not the act of killing. Finishing a downed animal with your knife is a bit closer. Cleaning and butchering it gives you some of the sounds and smells, but it is still not the same thing.

Slaughtering, killing a domestic animal, is different. It is more intense if you have raised the animal, named it, and it is a species that you like.

Rory never really liked sheep all that much, so slaughtering them does not bother him much. But he does like goats. And raises them. They are smart and wild, and have personalities. He learns more and it hits him harder to kill a goat.

Understand this: the point of this exercise is to hit yourself as hard as you legally and ethically can. See what you learn.

Legally—an animal, not a human; a food animal, not a pet; and one that belongs to you or you have permission to slaughter.

Ethically—you would learn more killing with your bare hands or making a botch of it with a knife, but any unnecessary pain is wrong. When you kill, under any circumstances, it should be as quick, clean, and painless as you can make it. That is the right thing to do.

Most of you reading this will never do this exercise. Those that do, your options are to raise your own animal or help out a friend who already butchers. It is nice to have small farmers for friends. It also helps because you will have someone with a proven method to teach you.

Rory has slaughtered with both a gun and a sword. Lawrence has done it with a gun.

That is the point, of course, and the importance of this exercise. Martial arts and self-defense, on one level, is the manufacture of cripples and corpses. Pretty that up if you have to, but if you need prettier words you have not come to terms with what you may need to do.

We could tell you what you might learn, about life, about weapons, and about yourself. But we won't. You need to do the drill, produce your own meat, and make your own discoveries.

Breaking the Freeze

You are in a fight for your life. You might think you know what you would do, or want to do, but in the heat of the moment you find that you can't pull it off. What if you freeze? Most people do when faced with extreme violence. Freezing is not moving when you are in danger. Sometimes it is involuntary, when adrenaline kicks in and you go into hardwired-freeze mode and cannot do anything. Sometimes it is tactical; you choose not to move because it is your best option for the moment such as taking cover during a gunfight. Sometimes, in the midst of a freeze, you honestly cannot tell if you can't move or just don't want to.

Perception under extreme stress is altered—both your senses and your perception of time. Some people, who think they froze in combat, were only frozen for a fraction of a second. They just remember it as a very long time. Or they think they are moving in slow motion but were actually moving normally. Some folks who clearly remember doing lots of things actually stood there with a blank look imagining doing stuff. Personal reports of events, particularly freezes, are unreliable for establishing facts.

One of the reasons that freezing is not well understood in humans is that there are many reasons to freeze, many ways to freeze, and that each type has different implications. Some are easier to train away than others, some can only be minimized, some disappear entirely. Some freezes feel like freezes. Some do not. And some do not even register consciously. That's a tough one because in order to break the freeze, you must first recognize that you are frozen.

If you believe you should be doing something and you are not doing it, you are frozen. If you are taking damage or seeing someone else take damage but have a warm, comfortable feeling and hear a rushing noise like the ocean in your ears, you are frozen.

Recognize it. Acknowledge it. Say, "I'm frozen." Out loud is better because it reminds you that you can affect the world. It is easy to say stuff in your head and not do it. Then tell yourself to do something. Anything. Scream, hit back, run, whatever. Say it and do it. Then tell yourself to do something, again, maybe even repeat the same action. And do it.

Recognize you are frozen. Make yourself do something. And keep it up until you are moving and thinking freely.

This will give you the best chance to act.

Principles for Survival

Self-defense is really about awareness, avoidance, and verbal de-escalation more than anything else. It is a lifestyle choice. You may find that you need to keep away from certain situations, people, or places to remain safe. If your friend's big mouth keeps writing checks that you need to cash, you are probably going to have to ditch that guy. If your girlfriend thinks it is cool to put you in situations where you need to fight for her honor, you are with the wrong gal. (Yeah, it could be your boyfriend doing the baiting, but that's rare.) If you are in a crime-riddled neighborhood, you may have to move, even if it is a significant financial challenge to do so. If you caused a problem at a bar, even if it is your favorite hang-out, maybe you should not go back. Find somewhere else to drink. You get the idea…

Unfortunately, even the best intentions do not always work, hence the need to move to higher levels on the force scale. When things get ugly, few fights are the same tactically, yet there are some overarching principles that tend to hold true. Keeping these strategies in mind can help you achieve a better outcome on "that day" should it arrive.

Be prepared

You wouldn't be reading this if you were not interested in defending yourself, but it is not just a paper exercise. Keep your training current, your skills up to snuff. Many folks earn their black belt and then slowly stop practicing over time. It is sorta like riding a bike; you never totally lose what you have learned, but if you're out of shape or simply have not hit the training floor in a while, you will be at a disadvantage if things go awry on the street. Practice is both mental and physical. We have talked a lot about mindset here and that is critical too.

If you carry a weapon, make sure you are proficient with it. And that you can get to it expeditiously. One of the challenges of concealed carry is that what you wear can affect your ability to get at your weapon. You may not have time to deploy it in a confrontation anyway, but make sure that you are not dressed in such a way that it makes it any harder to do so than necessary.

Justification is vital, being able to articulate why you had to do what you did, especially at the higher end of the force continuum. There are drills for that in here. You have practiced 'em right? You know I.M.O.P by now too. But it's a really good idea to go beyond what we've written. Massad Ayoob's *Judicious Use of Deadly Force* video is excellent. Watch it. Remember it. That is the kind of information that can keep you out of prison.

But that's not enough.

Spend time learning the intricacies of the laws where you live and work. The problem is that situations can change from location to location, even within the same state (or county). A knife that is legal to carry in King County, for example, may not be in the city of Seattle, despite the fact that Seattle is in that county. What is generally legal in New York State may not be in New York City.

It is unlikely that you can go beyond having a working-level understanding of this stuff on your own, and you should never represent yourself in court. Hopefully you'll never need professional counsel, but it's important to know someone who can represent you, particularly if you carry a weapon on a regular basis. Keep your attorney's information in your wallet, right next to your concealed-weapons permit (or concealed-pistol license, or whatever they call it in your area). The Armed Citizens Legal Defense Network (www.armedcitizensnetwork.org is a good resource for helping you find someone who specializes in this area of the law.

Preparedness starts well before the shit hits the fan, but that's not enough. Not by a long shot. You need to survive the fight. Then you need to manage the aftermath and win that too.

Don't get hit

Don't be there. Seriously. Do your best to avoid situations that are likely to lead to violence; you will live longer that way. If situations do go bad and you can withdraw or flee, that should be the first priority. After all, if you are not there you cannot get hit. And you won't be arrested. Or sued. Or have a whole host of bad things happen to you.

Taking damage sucks. The first person to be forcefully struck is at a severe disadvantage in any fight. This is especially true in armed confrontations. If you have been stabbed or shot, you may not be able to recover in time to keep from being hit again and again.

If you must engage an armed aggressor in combat, end the fight as quickly as possible to increase your chance of survival. Getting off line is important in any fight, but it is critical if the other guy is armed. It makes you much harder to hit. Doing so in a manner that precludes continuance of the attack or at least affords you the opportunity to counterstrike is paramount.

> My most successful tactic when entering a cell solo on a combative inmate was to step in deep just to the outside of the threat's lead foot while making a pass-parry motion with his own lead arm. Too many words. Basically, when all was said and done, almost every time a threat swung, he suddenly found the untouched officer slightly behind him and in full control.

Use movement to control the fight, removing options and initiative from the threat's arsenal. You cannot stand there and slug it out with an armed assailant. Even if you have a weapon yourself, playing "tank" with an adversary is always a bad idea.

The farther you are away, the harder you are to hit. If all he has is hands and feet, distance alone can keep you safe. If he has a weapon, you will need to use cover and concealment where possible too. Cover keeps the other guy's weapon from being able to reach you, say a concrete wall to stop a bullet. Concealment makes it hard for him to see and target you. Sticking with the firearms example, an interior sheetrock wall will not stop most bullets, but it does make it hard to aim accurately.

Embrace the pain

If you have been attacked, chances are pretty good that you were already hit too. You would not be operating at Level 6 if you were winning. You are likely facing a weapon, outnumbered, or both. Beyond avoiding the other guy's attack and minimizing the damage you take from the initial contact to the extent possible, your first countermove needs to either be fatal or severely disabling. The fight must be as short as possible. More so if you are already injured. No matter how much it hurts, keep fighting.

Most confrontations end with psychological damage, not because a combatant cannot physically continue. You already know that. The challenge is that at Level 6 you cannot stop until the other guy is no longer a threat. **While martial artists tend to hit harder than your average thug, a seasoned street fighter can hit harder than most black belts have ever felt.** In part this is due to the ubiquitous use of safety gear in sparring. Regardless, these safety precautions can put you at a disadvantage in a fight. In order to survive, you must be prepared to ignore the pain while mercilessly counterattacking your assailant. The "finding your limits" drill described above can help with that.

Pain is good, sorta, it lets you know you are still alive. That does not mean you want to take any more than is necessary. Nevertheless, if you embrace your pain and fear, it can serve to urge you on. Refuse to give up. Think about who you are fighting for beyond yourself—your spouse, your kids, your parents, your friends, and those who rely on you. What will happen to them if you do not survive?

If one's heart is in a fight, strikes to non-vital areas can have little effect at least not immediately. We have given all kinds of examples of that already. To put it another way, there is plenty of time to deal with pain after a battle is concluded.

During the fight, either do your best to ignore it completely or, if you are unsuccessful, use your pain as a reminder that you are still alive and still in the fight. Never stop until you have disabled your opponent and have escaped to a safe location. Then, and only then, can you afford to worry about how much it hurts. And get medical help.

Watch for weapons

An estimated 70 percent of adult males carry a knife or multi-tool on a regular basis in the United States. While most are law-abiding citizens who use these knives as the tools they are intended to be, the presence of a weapon changes everything in a fight. The end result of contact with a knife, whether in the hands of a pro or the hands of a punk, is the same. Anyone can cripple or kill you quite easily with a blade. It takes no special skill or training. Statistics show that, on average, someone is maimed or killed with one every two minutes in the United States.

Even if a fight initially begins with fists and feet, that is no guarantee that someone will not pull a weapon at some point during the confrontation, especially if they feel that they are about to lose. Be especially cautious if you face up to someone who leaves the scene, and then later returns. In most cases, you should be long gone by the time this could happen, assuming your situational awareness is halfway decent. There are thousands of cases each year in the U.S. where the loser of a bar fight subsequently retrieves a weapon from his vehicle, and then returns to seek retribution against the winner.

Although all violence is bad, armed assaults are far more dangerous to the victim than unarmed ones. According to the Bureau of Justice Statistics, while crimes of non-lethal violence committed with or without weapons were about equally likely to result in victim injury (approximately 25 percent), armed assaults are 3.5 times as likely as unarmed encounters to result in serious injuries. It's damnably hard to kill someone without using some type of implement. In fact, 96 percent of all homicides involve use of a weapon and nearly two million citizens are attacked with one every year.

Situational awareness is your first line of defense. Scan everyone that approaches you, especially if his hands are not in plain sight and you sense a potential confrontation. Look everywhere, but pay particular attention to the hands and waistline. A man wearing a fanny pack is frequently concealing a firearm within it, especially when there is a cord or tab sticking out from between the zippers. Almost anyone can conceal a weapon beneath a loose T-shirt, but you may be able to spot the telltale profile if you are paying attention. Experienced knife fighters never show their blade until they have already cut you with it. The clue with them is when they grab you with the off hand to immobilize. Even if you do not see a weapon in an adversary's hands, never assume that he does not have access to one.

This may sound paranoid, but unless you have personally searched an individual, it is a good idea to assume that he has a weapon at his disposal—hidden in a sleeve, hanging around his neck, stuffed inside a boot, strapped to his hip, tucked in a pocket, or otherwise available.

Because almost anything can be used as an improvised tool, be wary of anything within an attacker's reach as well.

You should not become obsessed about weapons, yet a healthy suspicion of those around you, particularly if they are acting unusually, and refined awareness of where and how weapons may be hidden are important for your survival. Listen to your gut. If something feels wrong, pay closer attention. Also prepare to act if you need to.

Cheat

Cheating is a time-honored tradition when it comes to a fight. If you practice a traditional Asian martial art such as karate or *iaido*, you probably know that the initial predatory stance of your *kata* (forms) is an invitation. This posture baits the adversary by offering up an opening. If you know where he is going to attack, it is easier to counter. In practical reality, the invite is not quite that stylized, but it is there nevertheless. It helps you win.

The same thing holds true today. No one wants a fair fight, least of all a predator who is looking to make a quick profit at your expense. Street fights are not duels, certainly not at Level 6; they are assassination attempts. Since weapons and numbers tend to tilt the odds in the other guy's favor, you need to be prepared to do just about anything in order to survive. There are many "rules" in a street fight. There are laws, of course, and physics, and all of your social conditioning, and the particular customs and taboos of fighting that every place has... All of them have consequences if violated, and, except for physics, all are in somebody's head.

Never underestimate an enemy. In a brawl, anyone is capable of just about anything—sucker punching, hair pulling, eye gouging, and spitting are commonplace. Throwing dirt in his eye, striking him in the groin, or deploying makeshift weapons are all acceptable tactics so long as the level of force is justified. The higher the stakes, the more you need to cheat. It's your life that is on the line.

An old con was showing me, as a rookie officer, how he read people. The old con pointed at one of our more seasoned officers.

"I wouldn't fight him." I raised an eyebrow. The officer was small, white-haired, not in particularly good shape.

"He's not strong," the con explained, "and he's not fast and he'd gas out early and he knows it. Young cops will fight you. Old cops are too lazy. They just kill you."

You might try to do something that is out of place, unexpected, loud, or disgusting. Anything that surprises an opponent can aid your defense. One of the best examples of this that Lawrence has seen was when two male fighters were tangled up; one leaned forward, planting a wet, sloppy kiss on the other's nose and then kneed his opponent in the groin as he instinctively flinched away from the kiss. Sure, that is not Level 6, but it does make a point. Even a properly delivered shout can momentarily startle or freeze an adversary leaving him vulnerable.

Anyone who attacks you thinks that he can win. He has almost certainly done so before. He (or she) may not look especially dangerous, but your attacker absolutely always has a bag of dirty tricks to use against you. Otherwise, he would not seek to fight you.

Once someone has assaulted you, never believe anything they say. A bad guy is by definition bad. He will lie, cheat, manipulate, and do anything else he can think of to trick you off guard. Much like he wants to avoid yours, you cannot afford to fall for your adversary's dirty tricks either. Be mindful of this.

Expect the unexpected

By definition, a threat is dangerous. He has almost certainly ambushed and possibly even killed someone else before attacking you. No matter what your rank or experience, do not assume that you are more skilled or better trained than your adversary. Consistent, high-quality training is the best way to ensure that you will have the skills and confidence necessary to prevail, but it does not necessarily prepare you for all the unpredictable things the other guy might do. Be prepared for anything, never letting your guard down until the confrontation is completely over and you have escaped to safety.

That preceding paragraph is one of those things that is both 100 percent true and 100 percent bullshit. Skill and high-quality training and all that are important and do give confidence, but the essence of an assault is the unpredictability and the extreme position of disadvantage. You do not just need skill, training, practice, and confidence in being able to evade attacks and hit hard. You need skill, training, practice, and confidence in recovering when something hard smashes into the back of your head while you are bent over and slammed into a wall with one of your knees not working.

Internalize this truth: Whatever skill and experience you have is exactly what it is. No more, no less. An experienced violent criminal has skill, practice, and experience at putting you in a position of disadvantage and completely dominating you or destroying you. UNLESS you have equivalent experience and practice at *recovering* from a position of extreme disadvantage, the attacker has an almost insurmountable edge.

Remember the earlier section "Situational awareness during a fight"? You might want to go over that section again, this time through the lens of Level 6. You need to be mentally and physically prepared to fight or continue a fight at a moment's notice. Always keep the threat in sight until you can safely disengage and escape. Even if your blow knocks an adversary to the ground, remain alert for possible continuation of his attack until you are out of range.

Situational awareness is critical. You cannot afford to be caught by surprise; that's a good way to die. Street attacks can involve multiple assailants. When multiple predators work together, it is reasonable to expect that they may be seasoned fighters who know how to take a blow and shrug off pain. Be mindful of additional assailants and be prepared to continue your defense as long as necessary. Remain vigilant until you are certain that your adversary is no longer a threat and that no one else is prepared to take up the battle on his behalf.

If you are facing multiple opponents, keep in mind that breaking out of a group is physically, mentally, and tactically completely different than fighting a group. If you fight or even defend in place, you will lose. You must fight to the goal and the goal is to escape.

There is no time for analysis in a fight. Do not get too locked into a plan. If the first thing you try fails, move on to something different. Immediately. Focus on the "now," reacting to whatever the threat does without thinking overmuch. Scenario training, such as the free-for-all drill we outlined above, can really help with this. The more strange stuff you've seen, the easier it is to respond to something unexpected in the heat of the moment.

Always keep your goal in mind; if you're fighting to escape don't get caught up in anything contrary to that. As soon as you get a clean opening, run.

Yell for help

Don't just yell, articulate. The word "help" is overused and often ignored, so screaming something along the lines of, "Oh my god, don't kill me with that knife" works a hell of a lot better. Not only may this tactic have a better chance of attracting the attention of a possible rescuer than generally yelling for help, but it also demonstrates for potential witnesses that you are, indeed, in reasonable fear for your life should you end up killing your attacker in self-defense. This tactic not only gets attention but also creates witnesses who may be sympathetic to your cause. After all, if you stumble across a fight in progress, there is no way of knowing who the bad guy is without extra information.

Creating witnesses can be nearly as important for your long-term well-being as defeating your adversary is for your survival. We live in a litigious, legalistic society, one in which information is ubiquitous and media judgment hasty and frequently severe. Beware of what you say and do. Always assume that your actions will be captured on videotape and reviewed before a judge or jury. Since a fundamental tenet of judicious use of force under the law is fear for one's life, your actions must demonstrate appropriate fear and actual jeopardy before you take violent measures in self-defense.

Attracting attention to your plight not only helps justify your actions in the eyes of the law, but it also helps eliminate the privacy that most law breakers desire while they commit their crimes. A predator who is winning may bugger off simply because he is afraid that he is about to get caught. While yelling for help may or may not spur a rescuer to intervene, there is very little downside in highlighting your peril.

Manage the aftermath

Once you reach Level 6, the fight itself is only the beginning. There are a host of other consequences to address, including medical triage, dealing with psychological trauma, interacting with law enforcement, and navigating the legal system, to name a few.

If a weapon was involved, you may be seriously injured without even knowing it. In most cases, you will not immediately feel pain because of the analgesic effects of an adrenaline rush. Consequently, you could be badly mauled, winding up with broken bones, severe bleeding, or other horrific injuries. Check yourself over to find out. Depending on where the event took place, you may have to tend the injuries yourself until professional help can arrive. Once you have treated your own life-threatening injuries, you might consider treating your adversary's too. It's not required by any means, but it does generally play well in court.

Anything you live through can be a good lesson as long as you learn something from it. If you are an average guy or found yourself hopelessly outmatched, you may be less traumatized by losing a fight than if you considered yourself a real "fighter" yet got beat down nevertheless. Wait a few days to regain your emotional equilibrium, dispassionately evaluate your objectives, and then figure out what, if anything, you should do differently in the future. It is perfectly normal to experience grief and anguish after traumatic events. Exposure to highly stressful experiences may lead to serious psychological trauma, however. Symptoms can occur whether you win, lose, or even witness a violent encounter. If you have been involved in an altercation and experience recurring emotional effects for more than a few days, it is a good idea to consider professional counseling to facilitate a healthy recovery.

Traumatic situations are frequently associated with critical-incident amnesia. The greater the stress, the greater your potential of experiencing memory problems. Although you may not remember much about a traumatic incident right after it occurs, you should experience significant memory recovery after a good night's sleep. This recovery period is important when dealing with the police. **Do not make stuff up; it will be used against you in court.** Do not guess, either, or try to fill in the blank spots in your memory. Retain your composure and conduct yourself in a mature manner at all times when dealing with officers who respond to the incident.

Expect to be arrested, even if you are completely innocent. Don't expect the cops (or press or anyone else) to pin a medal on you for being a hero. First responders need to control the situation; they can sort out exactly what happened and decide whether or not to press charges later on. Safety is their priority. A confrontational attitude will do you no good. You have a right to remain silent; in most cases it is best to use silence until you are represented by counsel.

The average person is woefully unprepared to defend himself in court. You want someone fully committed to win your case. You may be facing both criminal and civil litigation with your freedom, your job, your house, your relationships, and your money on the line. Find the best attorney you can afford and rely on his or her counsel. If you carry a weapon, it's a really good idea to have someone on retainer and carry their number with you in case you need to use it.

Putting it in Context

So far...

We're two thirds into the section on lethal force and we have not told you HOW to do a damn thing. That is deliberate. Any six-year-old with a butcher knife from the kitchen can kill someone. What a six-year-old is not prepared for is what that means. In all likelihood, neither are you.

We've spent two thirds of this section trying to get you to understand what we are really talking about here. It probably has worked for maybe five percent of you. The other 95 percent are perfectly happy with their fantasies...

And really, that's just the social context that a six-year-old does not understand. The physical context of self-defense is completely alien to most trained people's comprehension. Have you ever been hit, had your bell really rung? Maybe a good concussion? Start from there, but there is no pause after the hit, just more damage and you cannot see the guy because he is probably behind you and at least some of the damage is coming from your head bouncing off the wall or maybe it is the floor by now and maybe one of your arms will not work and you realize that you do not know who is hitting you or how many or with what and the blood in your eyes is starting to taste funny.

This is where physical self-defense STARTS. This is where you begin. If you haven't practiced your martial skills from here, baby, you probably won't be able to. Nighty night...

Targeting

This is probably going to surprise you, given some of the things we've written earlier, but killing people is not physically all that hard. There are targets on the human body that can reliably take someone out. Quick. The trouble is, like at Level 5, **they are easiest to hit when you are the bad guy**. Take the rear-naked strangle (or *hadaka jime* or vascular-neck restraint or whatever you want to call it).

You get behind the guy, wrap your forearm around his throat (careful to keep pressure on the forward sides of his neck, not the front), and then lever his head into the pressure.

It's a good technique. It is reliable. It puts people down by cutting off blood to the brain (or, technically, blood return from the brain). It does not matter how big the guy is, how crazy, or what drugs he has taken. If the technique is good, he will go out.

In a tournament, you let off as soon as he loses consciousness and he will be up and ready for his next match in a few seconds. Hold it for a minute or so, on the other hand, and you will cause permanent brain damage. Somewhere around four minutes, death. That is why it is considered lethal force in most jurisdictions: properly done, the technique is very safe, but held a little too long it is "readily capable of causing serious physical injury or death."

So, here is the problem: If you can get behind the guy, why can't you escape? If you can get the control to put on a naked strangle, how do you justify deadly force? Again, this is a quiz for you. We know the answer.

Think about it: To justify the naked strangle, you should be able to justify shooting the same person in the back.

Being able to articulate why you did what you did is critical. What was it about the situation that forced your actions? What did the other guy do? How did you know his intent? Why were you obligated to respond?

If Gary Fadden, who more than had I.M.O.P. on his side, was arrested and prosecuted for a capital crime, you can bet your sweet ass that you will be too. Or not. Maybe. It is prudent to plan for the worst and hope for the best. Remember that articulation drill we outlined in the "Legal Ramifications of Violence" section? Go back and read it again. And start practicing...

Most of the reliable Level 6 techniques you can execute unarmed have the same problem: You pretty much have to be the bad guy to make them work effectively.

Head

On March 17, 2010, Deerfield Beach High School student Wayne Treacy, age 15, was charged with attempted murder for attacking eighth-grader Josie Lou Ratley. The assault took place on the campus of Deerfield Beach Middle School in Florida, where Treacy is reported to have knocked Ratley to the ground and kicked her in her head with steel-toed boots. She suffered brain damage during the fight, was rushed to Fort Lauderdale hospital, and placed on life support. Two weeks later, she still could not breathe on her own and was expected to lose some use of the right side of her body after recovering.

Newspapers reported that Treacy had told a sheriff's detective that, "he committed this act of violence in retaliation for several text messages that the victim allegedly sent him earlier in the day in which she allegedly made fun of his deceased brother." Treacy's brother had committed suicide the previous year; Treacy found him hanging from a tree outside a Pompano Beach church in October.

Blows to the head are dangerous. Damage may be caused either by intrusion of bone fragments or foreign objects through the skull, or by causing the brain to bounce violently around inside. The former generally takes some sort of weapon while the latter can be caused by your empty hand. When the head is struck forcefully, damage may occur directly under the impact site (coup), or it may occur on the opposite side (countrecoup). When a moving object strikes the stationary head, coup injuries are typical, but countrecoup injuries are more often produced when the moving head strikes a stationary object because of how the brain bounces and ricochets within the skull case.

Violently shaking the brain can cause death, coma, or persistent vegetative state, but more often than not, it results in a short-term loss of consciousness followed by temporary (or long-term) headaches, dizziness, confusion, nausea, or vomiting. Amnesia, auditory abnormalities, or visual disturbances are possible. Other symptoms of a concussion can include slurred speech, disorientation, lack of coordination, unusual emotions, and reduced cognitive function. Damage can be cumulative, so multiple concussions over time are hazardous, something to consider if you do a lot of full-contact sparring.

The basal area, where the base of the skull connects with the neck, is one of the weakest areas of the head, hence easiest to damage. Fracturing the orbital arch is another possibility, but it is not always a fight-ender. Also, flatter areas such as the temple tend to transmit shock more easily than curved sections. This difference is important when it comes to contouring. Take the head-butt for example; hit flat places such as the temple with curved areas such as your upper forehead for best affect.

Getting offline is critical in a fight, particularly at Level 6. If you can get to the side, or behind an adversary, the head can be a great spot for delivering a countervailing strike (if you are behind the threat, justification can be a challenge, of course). You can use a punch, hammerfist, or elbow to target the head effectively, among other techniques. Do not support the head when striking though. Because it's highly unlikely that you can do structural damage to the skull without using a weapon, you will want the head to whip around to shake the brain as much as possible instead.

In a Level 6 confrontation, it may be appropriate to target the head even if the other guy is down. That means that using your knee or foot may not be out of the question here. Of course, using a weapon or smashing the threat's head into a solid object works well.

Throat

On July 31, 2010, Yeaseam Nelson, a 21-year-old student at Indiana University of Pennsylvania, broke up an argument between fellow student Mikhail Young and a woman by putting Young in a chokehold. Nelson held Young until his arms fell to his sides, denoting unconsciousness, then he released the hold and left the off-campus apartment where the altercation had taken place. When he returned later, he discovered that Young, 19, who had attended IUP's Academy of Culinary Arts with dreams of becoming a chef, was dead.

Nelson was arrested and charged with criminal homicide and reckless endangerment. At Indiana County Jail, Nelson reportedly told detectives, "I choked him out, I did it."

Prosecutors later dropped homicide charges after an autopsy determined that Young had died of a heart condition, likely the result of a viral infection. But, Nelson was still tried for reckless endangerment and aggravated assault. "Essentially, Young died of natural causes," District Attorney Thomas Bianco told reporters. "But, there was still a physical altercation."

Anyone who competes in a grappling art has almost certainly been choked out several times. Done properly it is relatively safe, particularly a carotid strangle that is released on time. Done improperly, it could crush the windpipe. When their air supply is cut off, people tend to freak out, going into a fighting frenzy right up until they succumb to lack of oxygen. Consequently, while law enforcement organizations used to teach "sleeper holds," it is now considered Level 6 in most departments (that still teach a force continuum). Likewise, in the courts. You need very strong justification to choke someone on the street. If warranted, a naked choke or lapel choke using the other guy's jacket or shirt may be applied.

Air chokes are another matter. When pressure is applied to the trachea, you can cut off the air, but like any other form of suffocation, it can take over a minute for unconsciousness. Between the pain (vascular strangles, by contrast, are relatively painless) and the feel of suffocation, most people will fight in a panicked frenzy to escape an air choke. Further, and worse, after you release the grip, a bruised trachea can continue to swell. The bad guy may die after it is all over even when you had no intention of killing him. This is one of the areas where you can see how sparring can give you false information. Tracheal chokes hurt worse than carotid strangles, so they often get a faster tap. A faster tap out in this instance does NOT mean the technique is more effective.

The windpipe is vulnerable just above the suprasternal notch. A blow or strangulation technique here can crush the cartilage of the trachea leading to suffocation and death. Even a finger jab or push can elicit severe pain. However, the throat is instinctively well protected from strikes by most people. Sort of. And that is one of the disconnects between sparring and infighting. Dropping the jaw protects the throat from strikes coming in from the front. It does not do as much from strikes sliding up the chest on the inside. If the other guy drops his chin and it becomes hard to target, you can often get him to open up by using an arm-whip, that is, capturing his forearm or wrist and snapping it like a whip. Pull from your hip and you will see his jaw pop up virtually every time. From there, you can target the throat with a bear claw, web hand, or potentially with an elbow strike. Shoot up along the chest for best success; it is harder to see and more challenging to block that way.

While a web hand may not cause much damage in and of itself, it is easy to follow up with a throw or takedown. After you make contact, continue to drive upward until his weight shifts onto his heels. Then twist and drop, slamming his head onto the ground with all your body weight. You can post your leg behind his knee too, but that is usually not necessary. Few people get back up soon after something like that takedown.

Upper (cervical) spine

> Mixed martial artist Zach Kirk, 20, suffered a broken neck and paralysis after landing head-first on the mat during a takedown attempt during a match on May 23, 2009. According to news reports, he regained some use of his arms after doctors replaced his fifth vertebrae with bone from his hip during surgery. Although the operation went well, doctors were unsure if would ever be able to walk again.
>
> Kirk was 2-0 heading into a matchup at the Mayhem Martial Arts show in Iowa, but the mishap occurred in the opening seconds of the bout. As Kirk attempted the takedown, his opponent tied up Kirk's arm in an attempt to stop him. They crashed to the mat together with Kirk's head taking the brunt of the fall. His body immediately went limp; the fight was stopped seconds later.

Damage to the spinal cord is very serious. The higher up the damage occurs, the more severe it will be. Cervical injuries, particularly those affecting the spinal cord near the top of the neck, can be fatal and often result in quadriplegia if the victim survives. The vertebrae, or bones that surround the spinal cord, are numbered from the top down, so you find C-1 where the top of the neck meets the base of the skull and then count down the neck toward the shoulders from C-2 through C-7.

With the exception of the cranial nerves, all motor and sensory nerves route through the cervical spine. In addition to complete paralysis, injuries that affect the spine at C-1 or C-2 can result in loss of involuntary functions such as breathing, necessitating mechanical ventilators or diaphragmatic pacemakers if the victim survives long enough to obtain medical care. In fact, any injuries above the C-4 level may require a ventilator. An injury at C-5 might leave shoulder and biceps control, leaving you with the physical ability to shrug. Damage at C-6 generally allows wrist control, but leaves no hand function. Injuries at C-7 can cause permanent problems for the hands and fingers. But, everything below the upper chest still does not work.

A person can have his neck (or back) broken and still not sustain a spinal cord injury. If only the vertebrae are damaged, the spinal cord is not affected. However, the spinal cord does not need to be severed to cause major problems. Even if the spinal cord remains largely intact, damage to it can result in loss of function. Beyond paralysis, other effects of spinal cord injuries may include inability to regulate blood pressure effectively, reduced control of body temperature (in part due to loss of ability to perspire below the level of injury), chronic pain, and loss of sexual function, among other effects.

The cervical spine may be an excellent place to neutralize a good grappler. There's a reason why the rabbit punch is illegal in every sport. It is also a good target of opportunity when moving off line from a charge where a sword hand or dead-arm strike can be effectively delivered. The neck is strong front-to-back, or side-to-side but not both directions at once. Consequently a pull/twist neck crank can cause serious injuries. One of the most effective ways to attack the cervical spine of a prone victim is with a stomp to the back of the neck, though justifying that may be problematic.

Targets we didn't list

A quick note about some other "lethal" targets. If you have been around martial arts for some time, you will have heard or read about a number of deadly techniques you can perform with your hands or feet. Maybe. We have probably heard of most of them as well. And they did not meet our standards. Below are some examples that did not make the list:

- The *nukite* (spear hand) under the solar plexus to disrupt—or even snatch out—the heart. Seriously? Disruption, bruising, pericardial tamponade might be possible, probably with a thrust from a baton. We do not really see it as being effective when normal human fingers are used. Feel free to prove us wrong. Practice up to a hundred fingertip push-ups, then jam your fingers into a *jari bako* (sand jar) a couple hundred times a day for ten or fifteen years...and tell us how it works for you, including the arthritis later.

- Lacerating the liver or spleen. If you break the ribs over either of these two organs, you can bleed them out and can cause death. Breaking the ribs over the liver is certainly possible, but exsanguination is usually fairly slow. But the ribs breaking in such a way that the jagged ends penetrate is random, unreliable, and not necessarily a quick fight ender, although an unlacerated liver shot has a decent chance since it hurts really, really bad.
- A series of acupuncture points in a specific order to cause death... Does it work? Our money says no. If the theory as presented by one of the more famous instructors is valid, it is impossible to survive a massage. Does acupuncture work? Sure. That is a given, but if the therapist needs to work with three to five points for up to 30 minutes apiece to get the desired effects, what are the odds you can hit the right combination for the optimal length of time, all while the threat is doing his level best to knock the shit out of you, in a fight? Even if it were to work physiologically, it would still require you to do precision targeting and advanced computations under stress. Might work for an assassin, unrealistic on multiple levels for self-defense.
- The coronal suture or bregma. On paper, it looks pretty good. Babies have the "soft spot" there where the brain is exposed with no skull protecting it. Directly under are the motor nerves...this should be the place, right? Unfortunately, by the time a bad guy becomes an adult, the sutures have fused and it is now one of the strongest areas of the skull. On top of that, both of us have been hit there multiple times. Lawrence got dizzy once. With an impact weapon or a hatchet (or if you wind up fighting very dangerous babies), this might be a target worth remembering.
- The center of the forehead. Just above and between the eyebrows the skull dishes in slightly on most people. Engineering-wise, that makes it seem like a good place to hit. Rapping it with a single knuckle does get that pre-dizzy feeling. The old documents of some systems consider this a lethal blow...we don't know. We are pretty confident that the required single-knuckle blow to that part of the skull might knock the threat out (or even kill) but would certainly break bones in your hand. Worth it? Big maybe.
- The pelvic gap. We do not know what ancient warrior monk or fifteen-year-old pimply kid fantasizing about warrior monks came up with this one, but we have been told that a "chicken-beak hand" upward into the "pelvic gap" (right on the bottom of the

pelvis, between the legs) can rupture the large intestine or colon and cause death. Seriously? The first thing we want to know is who, if anyone, is the sick bastard who actually tried this? And second, even if it works, what good is a lethal strike where the person does not die except for days later from a nasty infection?
- Stopping the heart. We have been told that a sharp strike to the center of the sternum done at exactly the right time can make the nodes (the electrical plexi that tell the heart when to beat) misfire and the heart stops. Again, anything that relies on microsecond timing is too random to count on. Further, considering the number of people who are hit in the chest every day in martial arts classes all over the world, if this were even a tiny bit reliable, people would be dropping to the tune of hundreds a year and we don't see that happening. Has it ever happened? Maybe. But don't bet your life on making it work under threat.
- Rupturing the bladder. We can see this one—a threat downs a couple of pints of beer; with his bladder uncomfortably full he takes a hit. That could be bad. But we do not have a reliable source for it happening or any idea how quickly it would be incapacitating. Most of the drunk-asshole scenarios are social, not predatory violence. The times when it is most likely to work are the times when it is least likely to be justified. Extremely adrenalized people tend to void their bladder (and bowels) anyway, making it even less likely to work in a Level 6 fight.

There are lots of ways to kill a human being. There are far fewer ways that an unarmed and surprised person can kill a human being, even fewer when the person who needs to act is at a complete disadvantage against a bigger, stronger, and better-positioned person. That's where you start for self-defense.

The basics do not change. From whatever position you find yourself in, you must get kinetic energy into the threat's body. That energy must induce shock by stopping oxygen intake or blood flow or damaging the brainstem that controls the blood flow. It is that simple, and making it happen under stress is very hard.

The seminar was about to start and I was talking quietly to the host and several of his senior students. The conversation turned to power generation. One participant, a very small lady, admitted she wasn't sure she could hit hard enough to injure a big man, so we started talking about different kinds of power, particularly whipping power versus structured.

"Show her. Use me." One of the guys said.

I begged off. A good whip develops a lot of power. I mean a LOT.

"No. It'll be fine. We can use your armor, we have a telephone book, and I'm pretty good at 'iron shirt'."

So we did it. A layer of the armor that I use when I am teaching entry teams, the Seattle telephone book, and an iron-shirt practitioner. What could go wrong?

The telephone book was high on his sternum, because I wanted as much structure as possible to dissipate the force, and that meant the larger upper ribs. The telephone book was pretty thick and the armor I like has a semi-rigid plate protecting the whole torso. Iron-shirt guy signaled he was ready. So I hit him.

He went down, completely limp. I've never seen anyone drop like that except an animal shot perfectly at the brainstem. For one frozen second I thought, "Oh, shit. The seminar hasn't even started and I've already killed somebody."

He started to come out of it as I was checking his pulse. Did his heart stop? No idea. But it was weird.

This is the thing you need to watch for. Weird, twilight zone stuff sometimes happens. This was a fluke. You tell the story, though, and people start to believe this is normal. In a few years, it becomes a technique…and we have one more story about how to kill a man with one shot that beginners believe with shiny eyes.

Remember: kinetic energy into the threat to disrupt oxygen, blood flow, or the control center.

Defensive Weaponry

There are people who are more than eager to teach you how to survive a shoot-out. Martial artists in every major city will take your money to teach you how to use a knife against another guy who has a knife. It is our belief that such training skips a few critical steps.

Everything in self-defense derives from the situation. The earlier you see it coming, the more options you have. You learn to avoid potential ambush zones or the places where a predator trolls for prey, and nothing bad happens. You see a developing dynamic and leave, cool. You miss the signs and wind up in an interview: You have a chance to handle it verbally and an opportunity to use the time to gather resources (like help or access to a weapon or improve your position), and each of those things also adds to your presence.

Which leaves most of the physical skills needed when they are least likely to work. Quit whining: that is why they call it "self-defense" and not "a walk in the park." If defending was easy and usually successful, bad guys would be out of a job.

> The key is not surviving a shoot-out or a knife fight. The key actually lies in getting enough resources on your side to turn it into a gun or knife fight.

Most people will never be attacked by a gun (or anything else for that matter). The one advantage of being attacked with a firearm is that the threat wants at least a little distance. Many people are surprised that shootings occur at such close range (usually less than two yards) and forget that almost every other type of attack occurs at a distance that can be measured in inches. A gun-wielding assailant may not give you time to draw, but unlike any other attack, he will likely give you space to draw.

There are three steps you must complete to defend yourself with a weapon under close assault: You must (1) access the weapon, (2) draw the weapon, and (3) use the weapon, all without being detected.

Two notes first: The threat is in the position of advantage. If he in any way knows or suspects that you are deploying a weapon, he can almost certainly stop you, and then he can punish you. We use "punish" to denote an excessively vicious attack intended to teach you or the bystanders a lesson. **Killing is killing. Punishing is intended to make you beg before you die.** He may even do this with your own weapon. Then he will claim self-defense and likely prevail because, after all, you are the one who brought a deadly weapon into it.

Secondly, you have to be able to use the weapon without injuring yourself. This may be harder than you think.

Accessing a Weapon

The type of weapon does not matter. The discussions that follow should apply, with slight adaptations, to knives, guns, *kubotans*, or even pens. Use your creativity and experiment.

How you carry the weapon is probably the most critical consideration in whether you will be able to access it. Does it require one hand or two? Can you access it with either hand or just with one? How vulnerable are you during the draw? How obvious is your drawing action?

Three considerations come into play—concealment, location, and retention.

The point of carrying a concealed weapon is that no one needs to know about it. That means that something hides it from his eyes. Most of the time, that "something" is also between your hot little hands and the weapon.

A weapon in a purse or a fanny pack may be damnably hard to access under attack. It will take two hands and will be pretty obvious.

A weapon under a loose shirt or jacket may be far easier to access. A weapon carried in an ankle holster…damn.

We had an arrestee come into jail, waiting in the 'chutes: "Sarge," he whispered.

I knew him (names have been changed), "What's up, Roberts?"

"Sarge, I'm carrying a knife. The cops missed it when they searched me. I don't want you guys thinking I snuck it in and kicking my ass."

He was still handcuffed. I was really hoping this wasn't like the time where the arresting officers had handcuffed a guy with a full-sized hunting knife between his hands on his belt in back.

"Alright, where is it?"

"In my left boot."

> It took me almost five minutes. Hunting knife in a boot with peg-legged jeans. Finally had to take the boot off and let him shake the knife out of his pant leg. No way would he have ever gotten that out to attack somebody.

Concealment ties in with location for one of the most critical aspects of access. You must be able to reach your weapon. You must be able to reach it from a variety of positions. You must do it in a way that, as much as possible, does not leave you vulnerable.

Ideally, it should be someplace where either hand can go naturally. That makes the centerline one of the best places to carry a weapon under these conditions. When you are curling up in a ball, taking boots from all sides, your hands will be over a weapon in the front of your waist band, but that is one of the toughest to conceal and not very comfortable. Everything is a pay-off between speed and risk.

If you carry on the hip, it may be hard to access seated in a car or when pinned on the ground, and if you carry at the small of the back, getting taken to the ground could leave you paralyzed from the waist down.

Shoulder holster is easy to access in a car, but with any cross draw, your hand can be easily pinned across your chest.

Ironically, a weapon holstered on the outside of the ankle may be one of the easiest to access surreptitiously in a ground brawl, but the inside ankle will be nearly impossible to access.

The third element that will dictate your ability to access a weapon is retention. How is the weapon held in the holster or sheath? Zero-level retention, meaning nothing is actually holding the weapon in other than gravity, makes for a very quick draw. It can also mean that when you lean back in your seat at a meeting, your hold-out weapon might thump to the floor for the world, including your boss, to see.

Single retention is a single strap holding the weapon in, usually snapped over the back strap or hammer. Double retention systems use two straps. Triple retention holsters use two straps as well as an internal block that locks into a piece of the weapon frame. Commonly, two straps must be undone and the weapon twisted or rocked in a specific way to un-holster a weapon from a triple retention (commonly called a level three) holster.

Whatever retention you use, make sure you can work the snaps with either hand, that you can un-holster while seated in a car, hunched over, on your back, or slammed into a wall. Practice the draw with someone grabbing you tight from behind and twisting your head up. If you cannot get the weapon into play, it is better not to carry it.

Even if you are carrying a weapon, you might not be able to access and use it in a crisis. Sometimes that means that empty hand is your only option. Sometimes, however, there are implements lying around that you can pick up and strike the threat with. Impromptu weapons are better than nothing at all.

Impromptu Weapons

I was cutting through the ravine behind my house. I'd hopped across the shallow creek that runs through it when they spotted me and gave chase. Predictably they caught me; it was, after all, three to one and they were older and faster. And they threw me into the muddy water. They'd done that before, but this time the guy whose foot I'd broken earlier that year jumped in with me. And shoved my face under the water.

And held me there.

It was only a foot deep, but I couldn't breathe. I freaked. The last clear thing I remember was finding a rock in the stream bed. My hand closed around it...and then there was just a red haze.

The next thing I knew someone was screaming, "Stop it, you're killing him." I found myself straddling the other guy, pummeling with the rock. There was blood everywhere. His face, my hands, the rock...everywhere. It's been almost forty years and I still remember the smell, the coppery tang of blood, the rotting loam of muddy earth, even the damp wool of his sweater, all of it.

Then I looked at my hand. I stared at the rock like it was some sort of alien, let out a gasp and hurled it away from me. Then I fled.

> Thankfully I was weak enough at the time that my blows didn't do anything worse than flatten his nose and shatter his cheekbone. If I'd been a year older, they very likely would have done much worse. Importantly, his buddies had the presence of mind to drag him out of the water and bring him home.
>
> I heard rumors that he missed a month of school. And had to have plastic surgery. But I honestly don't know for sure; I wasn't in junior high school yet. I do know that the bullies avoided me like the plague from then on.

Just about anything can be a weapon. Look in the trunk of your car (tire iron, jack, or fire extinguisher), by the side of the road (board, stick, or rock), at the table where you eat (bottle, mug, or steak knife), in your garage (hammer, shovel, or axe), or even at your desk where you work (hole punch, stapler, or phone) to find examples. Hot coffee and fire extinguishers can be especially useful as, unlike most weapons, they are extraordinarily difficult to block or evade. A fire extinguisher not only blasts a potentially disabling spray, but can be used as a truncheon in a pinch as well.

Heavy items like canes, tactical batons, flashlights, and even laptop computers can be swung with one or both hands to injure an adversary. A stout cane or short walking staff makes an excellent self-defense weapon, one that is legal to carry just about everywhere. There are certain martial arts specifically designed around combat canes, striking with the shaft as well as utilizing the hooked handle for grappling techniques. Similarly, tactical batons are designed for carry-ability and conceal-ability and are legal in many jurisdictions. While you do not always have to strike with these implements, control techniques performed by civilians using implements are often adjudicated in the same fashion as any other assault with a dangerous weapon, hence including them in Level 6.

You do not necessarily have to strike the threat with the weapon; you can also strike the weapon with the threat. This adds vehicles, walls, doorknobs, desks, stairs, curbs, handrails, and a whole host of other solid objects into the mix.

Drawing a Weapon

The drawing action itself must be concealed. If a bad guy is pounding on you and sees you going for your belt or digging in your pocket when you should be either fighting or submitting, do you think he'll ignore it?

The best way to conceal the action is to hit the threat. If you are carrying the weapon in a belly pouch, two hands are required to open it. An elbow strike would seem to put your hands right where they need to be, but think about it: If the strike is good, the threat's hands and attention will be drawn to the point of contact. Head and hands follow the pain. He will be looking right at your draw, and you still have zippers to play with.

A shoulder slam, though, uses your body to conceal what your hands are doing and gives him some impact to think about.

Biting is an ideal distraction. It is really hard to ignore. It focuses attention on your face, not on what your hands are doing. It can leave both hands free. Same with head-butts. The ideal distractive blow covers what your hands are doing, leaves your hands free, and focuses attention high, not low—unless you are trying to access something at upper chest or neck level.

Distraction is important, but that's just the first step. You still need to draw the weapon in order to put it in play. When adrenalized, that may be harder than you think.

Rory primarily practices knife work with a reverse grip. Not because it is better or worse or that was the way he was trained. He has noticed that under stress, he tends to grab like a brute. Even turning his hand down to draw a knife so it is in a standard grip is a little too slow, a little fine-motor. Since he knows that under stress, he is going to draw reverse grip, that's what he practices. Lawrence practices a standard grip. What works best for one person isn't necessarily right for another, you need to do what fits your predilections. Stress test it, then go with what works.

All of this leads to one of the necessary skills: the ability to recognize a potential weapon in your environment. If your hand happens to fall on a piece of brick, you do not need to access or draw it. You just need to recognize the gift.

Using a Weapon

Cut, stab, smash, or press a trigger, once you've drawn it you are going to have to use the weapon. It will be at a weird angle and distance, likely with most of your mobility hampered. With luck, you will have some mobility in your weapon arm, but possibly you will only be able to freely rotate your wrist.

Blunt weapons: Most of the smashing and swinging actions will not be available. They take more room than is common in an assault. Blunt weapon thrusts can do a lot of damage with relatively little energy. It does not take as much room to get power going, either. The problem is that very few of the close-range blunt-weapon strikes are fight-enders when the threat is enraged or insensitive to pain.

There is one exception that is devastating: the blunt weapon swung into the back of the neck can be very effective ground fighting or when the victim (that's you) is pinned up against the wall. The action is short and sharp, very much like trying to hit your own face with the weapon.

Edged weapons: When you do not have room to develop power, sharp is good. Push the point in and try to drag the blade out sideways. Bigger wound channels bleed faster, everything else being equal. Aim for the soft places, if you can.

Do this again and again until the threat stops or escapes.

With a sharp knife, do not expect to feel much resistance. It can be scary how easy it goes in. It will be wet and warm and have a scent—oxygenated and less oxygenated blood have different smells and guts or bubbling lungs even more so. Expect it and don't freeze. People freeze because things do not feel or smell or sound right. You may never have done this before; there is no "right" to compare it to (unless you have done the slaughtering an animal drill). Do what you need to do. Do not freeze.

If the threat springs away (some will, some won't) get and keep the knife between the two of you. Some won't even feel the blade; some will grip tighter. If he looks like he is still thinking about attack (and anything other than running away should be interpreted this way), keep the blade moving and be prepared to slash him off. Nothing is over until it is over.

We'll cover firearms later in this section.

Keep your verbals up. This is critical. The witnesses have just seen you stab someone. Make sure they know you're the good guy. "Don't kill me. Just let me leave. Please, somebody, call the police."

Blades

I noticed the scars on his arms and hands before he began the lecture. They could have come from something benign like working in a machine shop, but from the lightning speed with which he drew the weapon and the way his eyes blazed when it snapped open in his hand I knew that wasn't the case. He carried a blade like he'd been born with it.

"The first time I ever stabbed somebody I was 13 years old..."

If the way he moved hadn't already captured my attention, the way he spoke most assuredly would have. This was someone who knew what he was talking about, a "retired" street thug willing to share what had kept him upright and breathing long enough to get out of "the life." This was someone I needed to listen to.

While it is possible to run across a machete, sword, or even spear on the street, most law-abiding citizens who need a blade for self-defense will use a pocketknife. Most knives are actually designed to be used as tools, yet they can be deadly instruments too. They are popular, particularly in certain cultures, easy to obtain, and silent to operate. They are readily concealable, highly reliable, and do not take much special training to use to hurt somebody. They can be highly effective at close range, or even thrown at distances, not that we would recommend that. And they're easy to dispose of after committing a crime with one. Just sayin'...

Unlike guns, which can operate from a distance, knife work is up close and personal. It's ugly, messy, smelly, and downright horrific. Think about it. Are you prepared to stab as deep and as often as necessary to finish the job? By the time you are done, you will be drenched in your adversary's blood and viscera, you will smell his bowels as they release, and you will hear his cries as they fade to whimpers of pain and finally to the rattling gurgle of his last breath. Do you really want that? Using a knife to kill someone is not for the faint of heart. It's not something easily done.

Often considered "thug weapons" by politicians and folks in the media, if you use a knife on the street, you may have a tougher time in court than you would have had you used a gun in the exact same encounter. Most of the very same places that will not let you legally carry a folding knife do issue concealed-carry permits for law-abiding gun owners. It's a strange double-standard. Or maybe not. If you have seen pictures of both gunshot and knife wounds...

> We spent a day at a tactical briefing on terrorist sieges run by John Giduck, author of *Terror at Beslan.* The essence of the training was that there were people in the world who not only intended to target mass numbers of children, but who had studied our tactics specifically to increase the body count. If we ever were called in to deal with a terrorist siege, it would be local and the children under threat might well be our own.
>
> In the course of the day, John showed us videos of Chechnyan separatists executing Russian soldiers. Understand this: It was grainy video, there was no smell, it wasn't a child, and it certainly wasn't our fear: a child we knew. Yet one of the officers in the class fainted. I hope to god he wasn't a tactical operator.

Ironically while you cannot legally carry a blade over approximately 3½ inches in most jurisdictions, virtually everyone has a drawer full of eight- to ten-inch or larger "weapons" in their kitchen.

At the simplest level, there are two kinds of attacks with a knife—cuts and thrusts. Cuts generally produce more bleeding while thrusts can cause more serious damage, depending where you hit. Cuts can include slashes, chops, hacks, snap cuts, and vertical whips. Thrusts can include rakes, jabs, hooks, lunge thrusts, and loops. Cuts and thrusts are often combined as an opponent can feint with a thrust and then switch to a cut or vice versa with a simple flip of the wrist.

Everything just written is a dueling artifact. You do not parry and feint, and play some kind of game when you need a knife for self-defense. There is no flow. With gross-motor action, you slash at anything in reach to drive the threat back or, grabbed and trapped, you thrust again and again into any soft spot you can reach until the threat goes limp and lets go.

That is one of the beauties of wielding a knife. It's quick. And it's deadly. It really does not require any special training to use one. You could be a 300-pound tattooed biker or a 96-pound computer geek and be near equally deadly with a knife.

> *"I have watched people die because of knife attacks. The most memorable was my friend and bouncer colleague, Mike, who stopped a guy from stabbing him at the door. Instead of taking the knife away from the assailant, he cockily gave it back to him and kicked him out. At the end of the night that same person came back for his unfinished business. Mike started running after him into an alley and we quickly followed to help. When we got there, Mike was on top of the assailant who was unconscious. As Mike got up, I remember him saying, 'I got him good.' He walked about 20 feet and then fell to the ground where he died from internal bleeding. He'd suffered a collapsed lung and a severed artery.*
>
> *"Knives are serious and I dare say the most terrifying of weapons. I get upset when I see people practicing knife-defensive tactics with very little explanation. The most important thing to remember is that in training, one should never learn to feel comfortable with blades. This natural fear is what will probably save your life. Feeling comfortable with blades will make you lie really comfortably in your casket as this creates overconfidence that will lead to poor decisions. There's nothing wrong with learning these techniques, they do serve a purpose, but please keep in mind the reason why you are learning*

> *them. Use them as you would dangerous medicine; the same things that might save your life one day might also kill you the next. You might practice a technique perfectly a million times, but all it takes is the one you miss once to die from."*
>
> —Mauricio Machuca, a Montreal-based martial arts instructor.

Common targets that have proven lethal or severely disabling with blade weapons include the heart, subclavian artery (behind the collarbone), stomach, brachial artery, radial artery, carotid artery, femoral artery, axiliary artery, groin, and kidneys. Knife thrusts are generally more damaging than slashes, yet they also require you to move deeper into your opponent's target zone where he can easily reach you with his weapon, assuming he is similarly armed. If you have the *option* of moving in, it is not self-defense. It's stupidity.

Other frequent targets include the hands, wrists, and elbows, which may be cut at somewhat less risk of riposte. Such damage, while not immediately disabling, may convince an attacker to break off and retreat although you certainly cannot count on that happening.

You may not be the only guy carrying a blade, particularly in a Level 6 encounter. In essence, there are two different dangers from a guy with a knife. The first is a threat display, an extension of social violence. You see the weapon, he threatens to do something or wants to take something from you, and if you comply you might be safe. The other is an assassination attempt. This is predatory. Unless your situational awareness is exceptional, you probably won't even know that a knife is in play until you are cut with it. Perhaps not even then. It is common for stabbing victims to think they're in a fistfight until after it is over. Assuming they survive…

Bullets

Don't over-romanticize guns. A handgun is a nifty machine that throws a hunk of metal in a straight line. No more, no less. A .45 caliber bullet, unless it hits bone and sends fragments spinning, does just as much damage as driving a blunt 45/100 of an inch-diameter stick into the body.

Both authors have extensive training with handguns. Lawrence has attended a number of classes and shot competitively for a while; Rory has been trained as a tactical shooter for an entry team.

None of that means shit.

Shooting on a range is the skill of becoming steady enough that your nifty little machine can hit where you want it to. Trust us: Your gun is more accurate than you are.

Tactical shooting, and most handgun courses are based on tactical shooting, is the skill of crossing territory, possibly under fire, and getting accurate rounds on a target.

None of this is related to self-defense.

If you use proper stance and breathing and grip and sight picture when you shoot somebody, you are probably an assassin. Even combat shooters do not get all that. If you are using tactical movement and good cover to engage a threat, you probably should be using those same skills to get the hell out of there. Unless you are a military or SWAT sniper.

So what are the critical skills of self-defense shooting? Getting your weapon out and in play. Getting a round or two into a bad guy who is so close you cannot even really see him, while off balance, being knocked around and taking damage. Drawing the weapon and snapping off the rounds without shooting yourself. And, probably, immediate action skills because at that kind of range you can almost expect a semi-automatic to jam, since you will probably be touching the bad guy. At "normal" self-defense range, there is a real possibility that the muzzle blast will do more damage than the bullet.

Wounds

When it comes to bullets, ballistic performance (penetration, expansion, energy transfer) and wound trauma (level of physiological disruption), both affect stopping power, although shot placement is paramount. The only truly incapacitating targets are the brain and upper spinal cord. Even then, unless areas that control autonomic functions like breathing and the heartbeat such as the brain stem or thalamus are struck, headshots are not always fatal. A victim's chances of surviving largely depends on the areas of the brain that are struck, the velocity of the bullet, and whether the projectile exits the brain or bounces around inside the skull. If a bullet passes both hemispheres of the brain, the damage will likely to be much worse than if it affects only one side.

If the bullet misses the major blood vessels and ventricles, which are the cavities within the center of the brain that are filled with cerebrospinal fluid, the victim will usually have a reasonable chance of recovery if prompt medical attention is received. Because the skull is a confined area, however, swelling of the brain can prove fatal even if the initial trauma is not. Doctors frequently must remove part of the victim's skull during surgery. When swelling subsides, often weeks or months later, the bone can be replaced. And, of course, bullets travel through stuff so they often introduce bacteria or other foreign matter that can cause infection in the wound site.

Wounds to the heart, major arteries, and lungs may prove severely disabling if not fatal in rather short order. Nevertheless, these targets will not stop a determined attacker before he can hurt you. Similarly, damage to the head or neck that does not disrupt the central nervous system may prove sufficiently painful to stop an attacker. They are, however, generally not immediately disabling and can be shrugged off by a thoroughly committed adversary. The same problem applies to hits to the arms, legs, stomach, and groin; although a shot to the pelvis might render the threat incapable of moving or chasing you, it probably won't affect his ability to pull a trigger.

Headshots have the best odds of stopping a determined attacker, but they are damnably hard to achieve in real life. Many shooters are taught to fire twice to the torso first, followed by once to the head and once to the pelvis if the body shots do not work. In part, this approach usually works because the threat may be wearing body armor, which may not be discovered right away. Mostly, it is because it is really easy to miss when you are adrenalized. Aiming center mass not only makes you more likely to hit the other guy, but also increases the likelihood of bullets not passing through your adversary and traveling into innocent victims. Your bullet, your responsibility. No matter why you pulled the trigger.

Firearms

While handguns, shotguns, rifles, and carbines can all be used in self-defense, it can be very challenging to justify anything other than a handgun in court, save for in your home (or some places of business) where castle laws might apply. There are few good reasons to walk around with a long arm on the street unless you are in the middle of a riot or natural disaster. But, preclusion still applies. Why were you there in the first place?

> He is an up-and-coming lieutenant in a foreign service. He heard a story about something I did the week before and so he tracked me down to ask about some one-on-one training time. He wanted close-quarters handgun. Or knife throwing. Sigh. We went with the handgun. Four count draw, dry fire, firing from retention, moving and shooting, scanning. Because he was a leader, we also went into how to train: Faults to watch for, what would happen if his men ever needed to shoot as a team.
>
> At one point he threw up his hands and said, "I am so angry. Everything they taught us was wrong!"

What he had learned at his basic training were the fundamentals of pistol marksmanship. They weren't wrong, they were just incomplete. Beginners need to learn safety. It's stupid to accidentally kill yourself. They need to get some feeling for success and how the weapons work, so they become a stable platform. They learn grip and sight alignment and sight picture and breath control and trigger press.

They learn these fundamentals in a context that makes it easy for the instructor to monitor and easy for the student to correct—good lighting, good footing, hearing and eye protection, safety monitors, and not moving.

Those environmental basics are rare as hell in real life. Gunfire is loud and muzzle flash can be blinding in low light. Often not only is the footing bad, but it may be too dark to tell how bad it actually is. And you'd better damn well be moving unless you already have good cover. If you do have good cover, think about moving anyway, because the threat should try to flank you. And cover geometry can be counterintuitive—cover is often better the farther you are away from it. Said it was counterintuitive.

There are details that came at a price: When and how to fire from retention, why the weapon should be canted out when at retention—details that aren't on the beginning syllabus.

Combat shooting, whether raiding or counterambush, is a whole different animal than range training. Honestly, range training is probably closest to assassination skills, which aren't that useful for good guys.

But that doesn't make dojo or range training wrong. I go to the range. I practice my dry fire and failure to fire drills. When I have access to a good instructor, I go to my martial-arts classes. Nothing is wrong, but it is incomplete. So when I practice my dry fire, I know what I will see when the projectile hits flesh and I know what it will do to my mind and body, because I have experienced it. Once. When I go to classes, I know when I am practicing moving and when I am practicing breaking people. Often, in my experience, the instructor does not know that crucial difference.

It gets wrong for me in two ways: When the students insist that what they do is what there is. When they are taught that the real world changes nothing (one of the best grappling instructors in the world talking to a room full of LEOs: "No, we've never actually tried this in body armor and duty gear, but that wouldn't change anything." Sigh.), that there is a one-to-one correlation between the skills they practice safely with their friends on their nice clean mats and being ambushed by someone who uses violence professionally or is in a rage. The other "wrong" is when the techniques become centered around artificial aspects. Altering techniques for safety is inevitable, but when the altered technique becomes the "right" way and the effective technique becomes the wrong way, it doesn't work for me.

So I practice the pieces with as much awareness as I can of the totality, and the absolute certainty that there is a lot of that totality I haven't seen yet, knowing that I will inevitably fail and have to improvise.

Arguably, the most popular weapon on the street is the semiautomatic pistol. They tend to be lightweight, easy to carry, quick to reload by changing the magazine, and have more capacity than other types of handguns. They use the recoil or gas energy of spent rounds to automatically load another cartridge into the chamber until the ammunition is exhausted. If you "limp wrist" the weapon, it may not feed properly causing a jam, which could prove fatal in a firefight.

Another popular handheld weapon is the revolver. Revolvers are more mechanically reliable than semi-automatics, especially in close quarters, yet hold less ammunition, take longer to reload, and are frequently bulkier to carry.

If you are going to carry a pistol for self-defense, spend a lot of time at the range becoming familiar with your weapon, its sighting system, and how to manage the various malfunctions that might occur when deploying it in battle. Never forget, however, that targets do not shoot back. People do. At a regular range, you cannot practice moving and shooting, utilizing cover, or dealing with the adrenaline rush that accompanies a lead shower. Consequently, once you are reasonably proficient, it's well worth paying for a tactical course that lets you work on these aspects of pistol-craft. Additionally, become intimately familiar with retention techniques. The last thing you want is for your weapon to be taken away and used against you.

Shooting

The gun has to fire. It might not. Don't panic. With a revolver or some semi-automatics, a piece of clothing may have fallen under the hammer. If the barrel of many semi-automatics is pressed too hard against anything, the weapon is taken "out of battery," meaning the slide assembly comes back just enough that the hammer cannot fall. Get a little more room, possibly by striking the adversary, then pull back and try again.

This is also where all the complicated gear of a modern weapon can get in the way. You may be working at a weird angle that makes working the safety hard. Have you practiced working your safety by rubbing the weapon against your clothes?

You may have dropped and picked up the weapon with your thumb through the trigger guard.

You must know your weapon well enough to adapt.

You have to shoot safely as well. Yup, even in a fire fight. **The first rule of a close-quarters gunfight is DON□T SHOOT YOURSELF.** Chances are good that you will be shooting by feel, not by sight. Make sure that the body part you are pressing the barrel against is the threat's and not your own. Keep your hands out from in front of your gun. If you are going to shoot into the neck or head of a threat who is on top of you, slamming your head against the pavement, make sure you are not gripping his head on the other side—a flattened slug and bunch of skull fragments blowing through your hand won't help your piano playing.

You will touch the threat's body with the end of the barrel: The biggest part of the body you can find. By that we mean never go for edges. Whether you are shooting into the torso from the front, sides, or back, shoot to the middle of the torso, not toward an angle. If all you can feel is the leg, aim for the femur. For the head, right in the ear or through the nose.

Expect meat and blood to explode. Expect, like with a knife, for things to get slippery and smelly. If you have never fired a gun except at a range with hearing protection, you may be shocked by how loud the explosion will be, unless you don't hear it at all. Weird stuff happens in a gun fight. Be prepared for an insanely loud crash that will hurt your ears and make you feel like you have been hit in the head with a baseball bat. Expect to be burned and bruised wherever the muzzle pressure might have touched you. This is close-quarters work. It's nothing like shooting at a paper target.

Last thing: Unless you carry a revolver, expect your fancy pistol to turn into a single-shot weapon. At this range, someone will almost certainly have pressure on the slide, or be blocking the ejector, or the slide will not have room to move all the way back. Just expect the weapon to jam. If you can, the response is to put your off hand over the slide, slam the bad guy with your elbow backed by whole body torsion, and use that action to chamber another round. You will almost certainly not have room or time for a standard tap, roll, and rack.

Modifications, quality, and reliability

The New York Police Department did a comprehensive analysis of police-involved shooting incidents, evaluating some 6,000 violent altercations that took place during the 1970s. They found that officers hit their targets roughly a quarter of the time while criminal assailants made about eleven percent of their shots. This study dramatically demonstrated the effects of adrenaline. To look at it another way, highly trained professionals who nearly universally hit their targets in practice missed 75 percent of their shots during live fire situations. Criminals who presumably had far less experience handling firearms missed 89 percent of the time. Ninety percent of those shootings took place at distances of less than 15 feet. In fact, according to FBI statistics, 95 percent of officer-involved shootings occur at less than 21 feet, with approximately 75 percent taking place at less than 10 feet and a little over half at closer than five feet.

Many of the people who quote this study just assume that the degradation in skill is due to adrenaline. Many of these incidents were also by surprise and/or low light and/or with innocent bystanders nearby and/or on poor footing and/or under the conditions we have described, with a threat fully engaged in close-quarters battle. Fights happen in places, places (and conditions) that often affect the outcome.

These altercations happen fast, furious, and up close, oftentimes in grappling distance, so getting a sight picture can be awfully tough. Compounding this with adrenaline and adverse conditions, it is really easy to miss. This is where technology such as laser-aiming devices can sometimes be a help, assuming you can see where the dot lands anyway.

A major manufacturer came up with a neat idea, an integrated laser that's perfectly aligned with the barrel (unlike competitors who have an offset that throws your aim off at ranges longer or shorter than where it's been zeroed) and is easy to install without any specialized skill or tools. You swap out the slide release, pull out the guide-rod and spring, and replace them with the laser device. It takes maybe ten or fifteen minutes. Then you've got a brilliant aiming dot, one that's visible in broad daylight which could be a lifesaver in fast and furious encounters where you cannot use the weapon's sights to target the threat.

Great idea, right? I thought so. So I bought and installed one. It worked great for a bit, but broke after less than 250 rounds on the first day I used it at the range. The ring at the laser-end cracked, skewing it out of alignment. At almost the exact same time, the battery cap broke loose and could not be reset properly, jamming the slide. This wasn't a simple malfunction like a misfeed or stovepipe that's easy to clear; the weapon was rendered completely inoperative.

After fiddling with it for a bit I managed to get the slide to release. When I pulled it off the gun the battery cap popped out, flew four or five feet, and bounced another foot or two along the floor. I was able to find it easily enough, but could not get it to close and stay put after that.

Fortunately this all happened at the range. What if it had happened during an encounter where I'd needed the weapon for self-defense? Well, I'd almost certainly be dead right now. Yeah, DEAD. RIGHT. NOW. Because of the way the laser failed, the gun was rendered completely non-functional. Until the laser unit was removed and replaced with the original factory guide-rod and spring, it could not be fired.

No matter how well designed, mechanical devices fail. Clearly this one was defective to have broken so easily, but it illustrates how important it is to purchase quality equipment and maintain it in optimal operating condition. You must consider carefully any modifications you make to your weapon. If you replace vital components with aftermarket parts, even ones that are ostensibly upgrades, you may be asking for trouble.

One of the best ways to ascertain quality is to go to a range where they rent firearms and talk to the armorer there. While a normal person may only shoot a few hundred rounds a month, rental weapons can have upward of 30,000 shots per year run through them. If something is going to break due to use or abuse, armorers will likely know about it.

Consider a backup gun. Depending on the circumstances, it may be easier to abandon your primary weapon than to attempt to fix a problem during a fight, and draw a secondary firearm.

Wrap up

If you are going to carry a gun, you need to know the law in your area. You probably cannot legally carry a firearm into bars, schools, federal buildings, court houses, and (potentially) a host of other places. You also cannot leave one locked in your vehicle in many jurisdictions. This means that you'll have to plan your day carefully.

Shooting is a fine-motor skill. In your first encounter, training will only help up to a point, and even then not for most people. A good firearm is expensive. If you are going to become proficient with one, expect to spend a LOT more money on training and ammunition than you did on purchasing your weapon.

Level 6 Conclusion

Level 6 is about cripples and corpses. About you creating them or becoming one. It's not cool. It's not heroic. It's not like the movies. But you know that now. And hopefully you're a bit better prepared.

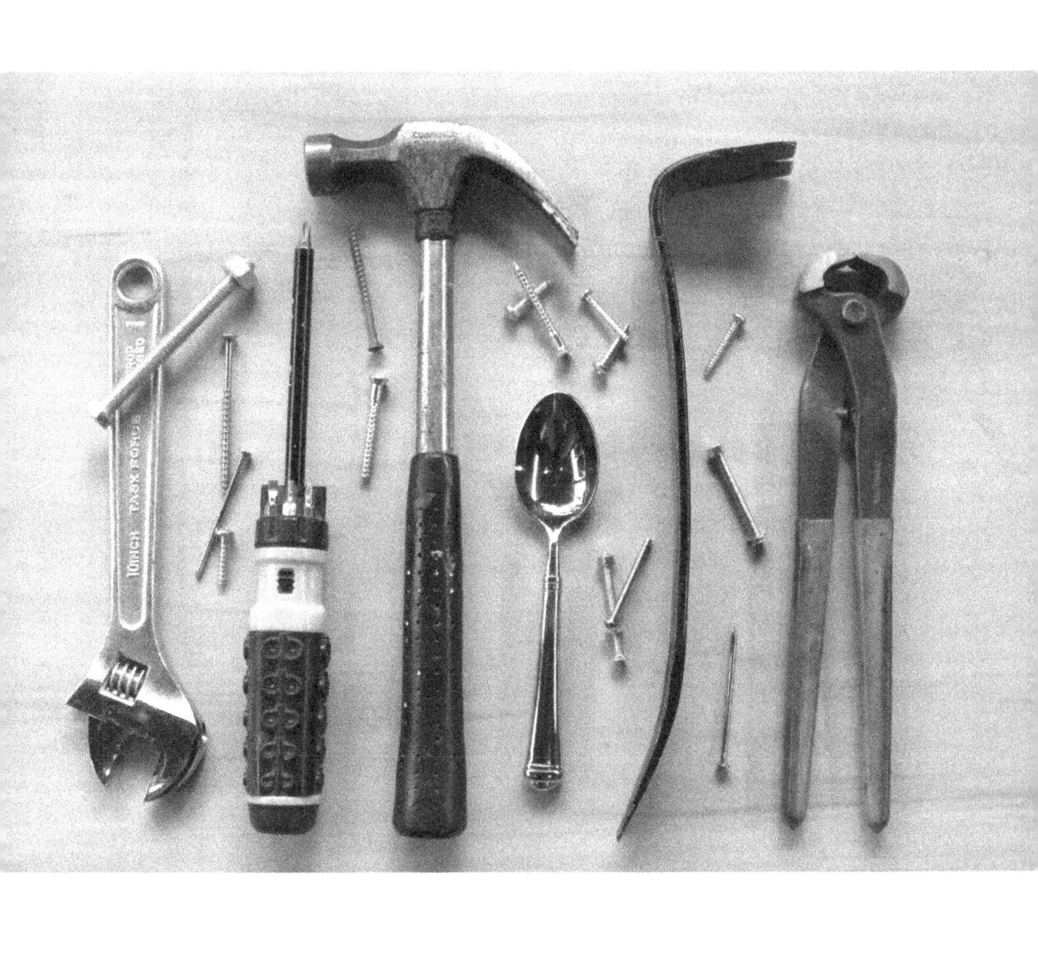
10INCH TASK FORCE

CONCLUSION

> "I study a complete martial art," the young man said, with decided emphasis on the 'complete.'
>
> "Really? Because that, to me, would mean that you study everything from avoidance and communication up through firearms and at least small unit tactics. We may just be defining things differently..."

We hope that if you have taken one thing away from this book, it is that conflict and violence are a very broad range of human behavior. The things that you may have to defend yourself against range from intimidation to murder and your appropriate defenses also must range from doing nothing skillfully to possibly taking a life.

Almost any martial art you can name focuses on one or at most two narrow ranges of response. MMA and classical jujutsu probably have the broadest range, training hard at Levels 4 and 5 and flirting with Level 6, but the most effective of the lethal techniques are banned or given lip service. It is not just that you fight with the techniques that you train, but you also ignore the techniques you have been trained to ignore.

That's a hole. It's not insurmountable, but it is a hole.

The lower-level force options are, for most martial artists, a much bigger hole. Almost all of us have been told it is better to run than to fight or that it is better to apologize and walk away...but who actively practices that? If you do not practice you WILL make mistakes and go with your social conditioning. Serious criminals thrive on your social conditioning.

Here is a scenario: A two-hundred-pound guy has promised that he is going to meet you at a certain place and time. At that time and in that place, he will beat you senseless or make you scream for mercy. Do you show up?

If it's self-defense, hell no. That would be stupid. If it is a match, you live for that shit. Get it? There are some fundamental strategies and assumptions that differ between any style of martial arts and self-defense. When the situation happens in an uncontrolled environment, you must be able to switch to the self-defense-centered strategies. You need to be able to act at any level of the force scale, from the highest to the lowest. You must be able to choose the appropriate level.

Spending a decade studying Level 5 and praying that any situation you might get into will just happen to be justifiable and solvable at Level 5...that's not a strategy. That's just stupid.

GLOSSARY

de ashi harai. Forward foot sweep.

dojo. Training hall ("place to learn the way").

gi. Traditional Japanese martial arts uniform.

hadaka jime. Rear naked choke (choke that doesn't require use of the opponent's clothing to work).

hakama. Skirt-like pants used in some traditional martial arts.

hijab. Traditional headscarf worn by Muslim women, sometimes including a veil that covers the face except for the eyes.

hiki uke. Pulling/grasping open hand block.

iaido. Art of drawing the sword.

irimi nage. Entering throw ("clothesline" takedown technique).

jari bako. Sand jar (traditional tool used for finger conditioning in classical karate).

kata. Formal exercise (a logical series of offensive and defensive movements performed in a particular order during solo training).

keffiyeh. Traditional Arab headscarf worn by men.

ko uchi gari. Small inner reaping throw.

koryu. Classical martial traditions (of Japan).

kubotan. A hard plastic or metal cylinder about 5 inches to 6 inches long that can be used for striking, pressure point manipulations, and control techniques.

kumite. Sparring ("to cross hands").

makiwara. Striking post.

nukite. Spear-hand strike.

osoto gake. Major outer hook throw.

osoto gari. Major outer reaping throw.

randori. Free sparring.

saifa kata. Okinawan karate kata ("to smash and tear to pieces").

sankaju (sankyo). Wrist lock.

sasae tsurikomi ashi. Lifting pulling ankle block.

sensei. Teacher ("one who has come before").

shiho nage. Four-direction throw.

sutemi waza. Sacrifice (momentum) throw.

tachi waza. Standing techniques.

tartan. Woven-cloth pattern denoting Scottish-clan heritage.

tori. Attacker (in a tandem exercise).

uke. Receiver (in a tandem exercise; also to receive or "block" a technique).

uke otoshi. Hand-drop throw.

yarmulke. Traditional Jewish head covering worn by men.

zanshin. A state of relaxed alertness ("remaining mind").

INDEX

BIBLIOGRAPHY

Ayoob, Massad. *The Truth About Self-Protection*. New York, NY: Bantam Books (Police Bookshelf), 1983.

———. "F You and Your High-Powered Rifle! The Gary Fadden Incident." *American Handgunner* (March-April, 2004).

Christensen, Loren. *Far Beyond Defensive Tactics: Advanced Concepts, Techniques, Drills, and Tricks for Cops on the Street*. Boulder, CO: Paladin Enterprises, Inc., 1998.

Christensen, Loren, and Dr. Alexis Artwohl. *Deadly Force Encounters: What Cops Need to Know to Mentally and Physically Prepare for and Survive a Gunfight*. Boulder, CO: Paladin Enterprises, Inc., 1997.

Consterdine, Peter. *Streetwise: A Complete Manual of Security and Self Defense*. Chichester, UK: Summersdale Publishers, 1998.

DeBecker, Gavin. *The Gift of Fear: Survival Signals That Protect Us From Violenc*e. New York, NY: Dell Publishing, 1998.

Grossman, David A. On Killing: *The Psychological Cost of Learning to Kill in War and Society*. New York, NY: Little, Brown, and Company, 1995.

Grossman, David A., and Loren Christensen. *On Combat: The Psychology and Physiology of Deadly Conflict in War and Peace*. Belleville, IL: PPCT Research Publications, 2004.

Jay, Wally. *Small-Circle Jujitsu*. Santa Clarita, CA: Ohara Publications, 1989.

Kane, Lawrence A. *Surviving Armed Assaults: A Martial Artists Guide to Weapons, Street Violence, and Countervailing Force*. Boston, MA: YMAA Publication Center, 2006.

Kane, Lawrence A., and Kris Wilder. *The Little Black Book of Violence: What Every Young Man Needs to Know About Fighting*. Wolfeboro, NH: YMAA Publication Center, 2009.

MacYoung, Marc. *Cheap Shots, Ambushes, and Other Lessons: A Down and Dirty Book on Streetfighting and Survival*. Boulder, CO: Paladin Enterprises, Inc., 1989.

———. *Fists, Wits, and a Wicked Right: Surviving on the Wild Side of the Street*. Boulder, CO: Paladin Enterprises, Inc., 1991.

———. *Floor Fighting: Stompings, Maimings, and Other Things to Avoid When a Fight Goes to the Ground*. Boulder, CO: Paladin Enterprises, Inc., 1993.

———. *Knives, Knife Fighting, And Related Hassles: How to Survive a Real Knife Fight*. Boulder, CO: Paladin Enterprises, Inc., 1990.

———. *Pool Cues, Beer Bottles, & Baseball Bats: Animal's Guide to Improvised Weapons for Self-Defense and Survival*. Boulder, CO: Paladin Enterprises, Inc., 1990.

———. *A Professional's Guide to Ending Violence Quickly*. Boulder, CO: Paladin Enterprises, Inc., 1993.

———. *Street E & E: Evading, Escaping, and Other Ways to Save Your Ass When Things Get Ugly*. Boulder, CO: Paladin Enterprises, Inc., 1993.

———. *Violence, Blunders, and Fractured Jaws: Advanced Awareness Techniques and Street Etiquette*. Boulder, CO: Paladin Enterprises, Inc., 1992.

Miller, Rory A. *Facing Violence: Preparing for the Unexpected*. Wolfeboro, NH: YMAA Publication Center, 2011.

———. *Force Decisions: A Citizen's Guide to Understanding How Police Determine Appropriate Use of Force.* Wolfeboro, NH: YMAA Publication Center, April 2012.

———. *Meditations on Violence: A Comparison of Martial Arts Training and Real World Violence.* Wolfeboro, NH: YMAA Publication Center, 2008.

Quinn, Peyton. *Bouncer's Guide to Barroom Brawling: Dealing with the Sucker Puncher, Streetfighter, and Ambusher.* Boulder, CO: Paladin Enterprises, Inc., 1990.

———. *Real Fighting: Adrenaline Stress Conditioning through Scenario-Based Training.* Boulder, CO: Paladin Enterprises, Inc., 1996.

Siddle, Bruce K. *Sharpening the Warrior's Edge: The Psychology and Science of Training.* Millstadt, IL: PPCT Research Publications, Inc., 1995.

Thompson, George. *Verbal Judo: The Gentle Art of Persuasion.* New York, NY: HarperCollins, 1993.

Wilder, Kris. *The Way of Sanchin Kata: The Application of Power.* Boston: YMAA Publication Center, 2007.

———. *Sanchin Kata: Traditional Training for Karate Power.* Boston: YMAA Publication Center, 2010. (DVD), 60 min.

ABOUT THE AUTHORS

Rory Miller

Rory is the author of *Meditations on Violence* (USA Book News—2008 Best Books Award Finalist; ForeWord Magazine 2008 Book of the Year Award Finalist), *Violence: A Writer's Guide*, and *Facing* Violen*ce: Preparing for the Unexpected*. His new book, *Force Decisions: A Citizen's Guide to Understanding How Police Determine Appropriate Use of Force,* will be available April 2012. His writings have also been featured in Loren Christensen's *Fighter's Fact Book 2: The Street*, Kane/Wilder's *The Little Black Book of Violence*, and *The Way to Black Belt*. He has been studying martial arts since 1981. Though he started in competitive martial sports, earning college varsities in judo and fencing, he found his martial "home" in the early Tokugawa-era battlefield system of *Sosuishi-ryu kumi uchi (jujutsu)*.

A veteran corrections officer and Corrections Emergency Response Team (CERT) leader, Rory has hands-on experience in hundreds of violent altercations. He has designed and taught courses for law enforcement agencies including confrontational simulations, uncontrolled environments, crisis communications with the mentally ill, CERT operations and planning, defensive tactics, and use of force policy. His training also includes witness protection, close-quarters handgun, Americans for Effective Law Enforcement (AELE) discipline and internal investigations, hostage negotiations, and survival and integrated use of force. He recently spent a year in Iraq helping the government there develop its prison management system. Rory currently teaches seminars on violence internationally, and in partnership with Marc MacYoung has developed Conflict Communications, a definitive resource for understanding and controlling conflict. Rory's website is www.chirontraining.com. He lives near Portland, Oregon.

Lawrence Kane

Lawrence is the author of *Surviving Armed Assaults*, *Martial Arts Instruction*, and *Blinded by the Night*, and co-author (with Kris Wilder) of *The Way of Kata*, *The Way to Black Belt*, *How to Win a Fight,* and *The Little Black Book of Violence* (USA Book News Best Books Award Finalist; ForeWord Magazine Book of the Year Award Finalist). He also has written numerous articles on martial arts, self-defense, and related topics for prestigious publications such as *International Ryukyu Karate-jutsu Research Society Journal*, *Jissen*, *Fighting Arts*, and *Traditional Karate* magazine. His work has also been featured in *Fighter's Fact Book 2: The Street* by Loren Christensen, and *Wicked Wisdom: Explorations Into the Dark Side* by Bohdi Sanders and Shawn Kovacich.

Since 1970, he has studied and taught traditional Asian martial arts, medieval European combat, and modern close-quarter weapon techniques. He co-hosts a weekly podcast with Kris Wilder at www.martial-secrets.com. Working stadium security part-time, he has been involved in hundreds of violent altercations, but gets paid to watch football. To cover the bills, he develops sourcing strategies for an aerospace company where he gets to play with billions of dollars of other people's money and to make really important decisions. Lawrence lives in Seattle, Washington.

BOOKS FROM YMAA

6 HEALING MOVEMENTS
101 REFLECTIONS ON TAI CHI CHUAN
108 INSIGHTS INTO TAI CHI CHUAN
ADVANCING IN TAE KWON DO
ANALYSIS OF SHAOLIN CHIN NA 2ND ED
ANCIENT CHINESE WEAPONS
ART OF HOJO UNDO
ARTHRITIS RELIEF, 3RD ED.
BACK PAIN RELIEF, 2ND ED.
BAGUAZHANG, 2ND ED.
CARDIO KICKBOXING ELITE
CHIN NA IN GROUND FIGHTING
CHINESE FAST WRESTLING
CHINESE FITNESS
CHINESE TUI NA MASSAGE
CHOJUN
COMPREHENSIVE APPLICATIONS OF SHAOLIN CHIN NA
CONFLICT COMMUNICATION
CROCODILE AND THE CRANE: A NOVEL
CUTTING SEASON: A XENON PEARL MARTIAL ARTS THRILLER
DEFENSIVE TACTICS
DESHI: A CONNOR BURKE MARTIAL ARTS THRILLER
DIRTY GROUND
DR. WU'S HEAD MASSAGE
DUKKHA HUNGRY GHOSTS
DUKKHA REVERB
DUKKHA, THE SUFFERING: AN EYE FOR AN EYE
DUKKHA UNLOADED
ENZAN: THE FAR MOUNTAIN, A CONNOR BURKE MARTIAL ARTS THRILLER
ESSENCE OF SHAOLIN WHITE CRANE
EXPLORING TAI CHI
FACING VIOLENCE
FIGHT BACK
FIGHT LIKE A PHYSICIST
THE FIGHTER'S BODY
FIGHTER'S FACT BOOK
FIGHTER'S FACT BOOK 2
FIGHTING THE PAIN RESISTANT ATTACKER
FIRST DEFENSE
FORCE DECISIONS: A CITIZENS GUIDE
FOX BORROWS THE TIGER'S AWE
INSIDE TAI CHI
KAGE: THE SHADOW, A CONNOR BURKE MARTIAL ARTS THRILLER
KATA AND THE TRANSMISSION OF KNOWLEDGE
KRAV MAGA PROFESSIONAL TACTICS
KRAV MAGA WEAPON DEFENSES
LITTLE BLACK BOOK OF VIOLENCE
LIUHEBAFA FIVE CHARACTER SECRETS
MARTIAL ARTS ATHLETE
MARTIAL ARTS INSTRUCTION
MARTIAL WAY AND ITS VIRTUES
MASK OF THE KING
MEDITATIONS ON VIOLENCE
MIND/BODY FITNESS
THE MIND INSIDE TAI CHI
THE MIND INSIDE YANG STYLE TAI CHI CHUAN
MUGAI RYU
NATURAL HEALING WITH QIGONG
NORTHERN SHAOLIN SWORD, 2ND ED.
OKINAWA'S COMPLETE KARATE SYSTEM: ISSHIN RYU
POWER BODY
PRINCIPLES OF TRADITIONAL CHINESE MEDICINE
QIGONG FOR HEALTH & MARTIAL ARTS 2ND ED.
QIGONG FOR LIVING
QIGONG FOR TREATING COMMON AILMENTS
QIGONG MASSAGE
QIGONG MEDITATION: EMBRYONIC BREATHING
QIGONG MEDITATION: SMALL CIRCULATION
QIGONG, THE SECRET OF YOUTH: DA MO'S CLASSICS
QUIET TEACHER: A XENON PEARL MARTIAL ARTS THRILLER
RAVEN'S WARRIOR
REDEMPTION
ROOT OF CHINESE QIGONG, 2ND ED.
SCALING FORCE
SENSEI: A CONNOR BURKE MARTIAL ARTS THRILLER
SHIHAN TE: THE BUNKAI OF KATA
SHIN GI TAI: KARATE TRAINING FOR BODY, MIND, AND SPIRIT
SIMPLE CHINESE MEDICINE
SIMPLE QIGONG EXERCISES FOR HEALTH, 3RD ED.
SIMPLIFIED TAI CHI CHUAN, 2ND ED.
SIMPLIFIED TAI CHI FOR BEGINNERS
SOLO TRAINING
SOLO TRAINING 2
SUDDEN DAWN: THE EPIC JOURNEY OF BODHIDHARMA
SUNRISE TAI CHI
SUNSET TAI CHI
SURVIVING ARMED ASSAULTS
TAE KWON DO: THE KOREAN MARTIAL ART
TAEKWONDO BLACK BELT POOMSAE
TAEKWONDO: A PATH TO EXCELLENCE
TAEKWONDO: ANCIENT WISDOM FOR THE MODERN WARRIOR
TAEKWONDO: DEFENSES AGAINST WEAPONS
TAEKWONDO: SPIRIT AND PRACTICE
TAO OF BIOENERGETICS
TAI CHI BALL QIGONG: FOR HEALTH AND MARTIAL ARTS
TAI CHI BALL WORKOUT FOR BEGINNERS
TAI CHI BOOK
TAI CHI CHIN NA: THE SEIZING ART OF TAI CHI CHUAN, 2ND ED.
TAI CHI CHUAN CLASSICAL YANG STYLE, 2ND ED.
TAI CHI CHUAN MARTIAL APPLICATIONS
TAI CHI CHUAN MARTIAL POWER, 3RD ED.
TAI CHI CONNECTIONS
TAI CHI DYNAMICS
TAI CHI QIGONG, 3RD ED.
TAI CHI SECRETS OF THE ANCIENT MASTERS
TAI CHI SECRETS OF THE WU & LI STYLES
TAI CHI SECRETS OF THE WU STYLE
TAI CHI SECRETS OF THE YANG STYLE
TAI CHI SWORD: CLASSICAL YANG STYLE, 2ND ED.
TAI CHI SWORD FOR BEGINNERS
TAI CHI WALKING
TAIJIQUAN THEORY OF DR. YANG, JWING-MING
TENGU: THE MOUNTAIN GOBLIN, A CONNOR BURKE MARTIAL ARTS THRILLER
TIMING IN THE FIGHTING ARTS
TRADITIONAL CHINESE HEALTH SECRETS
TRADITIONAL TAEKWONDO
TRAINING FOR SUDDEN VIOLENCE
WAY OF KATA
WAY OF KENDO AND KENJITSU
WAY OF SANCHIN KATA
WAY TO BLACK BELT
WESTERN HERBS FOR MARTIAL ARTISTS
WILD GOOSE QIGONG
WOMAN'S QIGONG GUIDE
XINGYIQUAN

DVDS FROM YMAA

ADVANCED PRACTICAL CHIN NA IN-DEPTH
ANALYSIS OF SHAOLIN CHIN NA
ATTACK THE ATTACK
BAGUAZHANG: EMEI BAGUAZHANG
CHEN STYLE TAIJIQUAN
CHIN NA IN-DEPTH COURSES 1—4
CHIN NA IN-DEPTH COURSES 5—8
CHIN NA IN-DEPTH COURSES 9—12
FACING VIOLENCE: 7 THINGS A MARTIAL ARTIST MUST KNOW
FIVE ANIMAL SPORTS
JOINT LOCKS
KNIFE DEFENSE: TRADITIONAL TECHNIQUES AGAINST A DAGGER
KUNG FU BODY CONDITIONING 1
KUNG FU BODY CONDITIONING 2
KUNG FU FOR KIDS
KUNG FU FOR TEENS
INFIGHTING
LOGIC OF VIOLENCE
MERIDIAN QIGONG
NEIGONG FOR MARTIAL ARTS
NORTHERN SHAOLIN SWORD : SAN CAI JIAN, KUN WU JIAN, QI MEN JIAN
QIGONG MASSAGE
QIGONG FOR HEALING
QIGONG FOR LONGEVITY
QIGONG FOR WOMEN
SABER FUNDAMENTAL TRAINING
SAI TRAINING AND SEQUENCES
SANCHIN KATA: TRADITIONAL TRAINING FOR KARATE POWER
SHAOLIN KUNG FU FUNDAMENTAL TRAINING: COURSES 1 & 2
SHAOLIN LONG FIST KUNG FU: BASIC SEQUENCES
SHAOLIN LONG FIST KUNG FU: INTERMEDIATE SEQUENCES
SHAOLIN LONG FIST KUNG FU: ADVANCED SEQUENCES 1
SHAOLIN LONG FIST KUNG FU: ADVANCED SEQUENCES 2
SHAOLIN SABER: BASIC SEQUENCES
SHAOLIN STAFF: BASIC SEQUENCES
SHAOLIN WHITE CRANE GONG FU BASIC TRAINING: COURSES 1 & 2
SHAOLIN WHITE CRANE GONG FU BASIC TRAINING: COURSES 3 & 4
SHUAI JIAO: KUNG FU WRESTLING
SIMPLE QIGONG EXERCISES FOR ARTHRITIS RELIEF
SIMPLE QIGONG EXERCISES FOR BACK PAIN RELIEF
SIMPLIFIED TAI CHI CHUAN: 24 & 48 POSTURES
SIMPLIFIED TAI CHI FOR BEGINNERS 48
SUNRISE TAI CHI
SUNSET TAI CHI
SWORD: FUNDAMENTAL TRAINING
TAEKWONDO KORYO POOMSAE
TAI CHI BALL QIGONG: COURSES 1 & 2
TAI CHI BALL QIGONG: COURSES 3 & 4
TAI CHI BALL WORKOUT FOR BEGINNERS
TAI CHI CHUAN CLASSICAL YANG STYLE
TAI CHI CONNECTIONS
TAI CHI ENERGY PATTERNS
TAI CHI FIGHTING SET
TAI CHI PUSHING HANDS: COURSES 1 & 2
TAI CHI PUSHING HANDS: COURSES 3 & 4
TAI CHI SWORD: CLASSICAL YANG STYLE
TAI CHI SWORD FOR BEGINNERS
TAI CHI SYMBOL: YIN YANG STICKING HANDS
TAIJI & SHAOLIN STAFF: FUNDAMENTAL TRAINING
TAIJI CHIN NA IN-DEPTH
TAIJI 37 POSTURES MARTIAL APPLICATIONS
TAIJI SABER CLASSICAL YANG STYLE
TAIJI WRESTLING
TRAINING FOR SUDDEN VIOLENCE
UNDERSTANDING QIGONG 1: WHAT IS QI? • HUMAN QI CIRCULATORY SYSTEM
UNDERSTANDING QIGONG 2: KEY POINTS • QIGONG BREATHING
UNDERSTANDING QIGONG 3: EMBRYONIC BREATHING
UNDERSTANDING QIGONG 4: FOUR SEASONS QIGONG
UNDERSTANDING QIGONG 5: SMALL CIRCULATION
UNDERSTANDING QIGONG 6: MARTIAL QIGONG BREATHING
WHITE CRANE HARD & SOFT QIGONG
WUDANG KUNG FU: FUNDAMENTAL TRAINING
WUDANG SWORD
WUDANG TAIJIQUAN
XINGYIQUAN
YANG TAI CHI FOR BEGINNERS
YMAA 25 YEAR ANNIVERSARY DVD

Printed in the USA
CPSIA information can be obtained
at www.ICGtesting.com
JSHW022207140824
68134JS00018B/902